Getting

to Know

the Troubled

Child

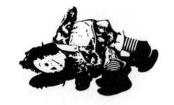

Getting
to Know
the Troubled
Child

DAVID H. LOOFF, M.D.

THE UNIVERSITY OF TENNESSEE PRESS

Library of Congress Cataloging in Publication Data

Looff, David H.   1928-
   Getting to know the troubled child.

   Includes bibliographical references and index.
   1. Child psychiatry. 2. Interviewing in
psychiatry. I. Title. [DNLM: 1. Interview,
Psychological—In infancy & childhood. 2. Child
behavior disorders. 3. Mental disorders—In infancy
& childhood. WS350 L861g]
 RJ499.L66   618.9'28'9075   75-43691
 IBSN 0-87049-190-3

To my wife, Glyndon, whose love through the years has supported many an endeavor. And to our son, John, and to our daughter, Mary, with love, admiration, and respect.

Preface

Troubled children—whether toddlers, preschoolers, school-age youngsters, or adolescents—present a great variety of problems for their families, their teachers, and those professionals who may be called upon to help them. The problems range from minor difficulties of adjustment to disturbances of crisis proportions. These frightened, shy, rebellious, sad, confused youngsters come from all walks of life in increasing numbers.

Once the decision has been made to seek help, usually by the troubled child's parents, teacher, physician or someone interested in his or her welfare, the child is referred to an individual specialist or to one of the public or private clinics or offices that handle such cases. Often the helping agency is one of the growing number of community mental health centers in this nation.

The first important task that faces us in the clinical setting is that of getting to know these troubled children and their families. We may be psychiatrists, pediatricians, social workers, psychologists, psychiatric nurses, mental health associates, or trainees in these fields—but regardless of our type of training and length of experience, we face the same problem. On meeting a child and his family for the first time, we invariably pose the silent questions: What shall I say to this troubled child? What can I do to gain his confidence? How can I reach him and his family in order to understand the reasons for his difficulties?

This book attempts to answer these questions. It is an elementary guide, designed to introduce the subject and provide some practical help in the establishment of good interview and assessment techniques for those in the mental health field, regardless of their specialty, who are just beginning to work with children. It may also, I hope, be read with profit by parents, teachers, physicians, in fact by any persons who seek to increase their sensitivity to the needs of children.

The book is, by design, a very personal one, being based on my experiences during the past fourteen years as a clinical child psychiatrist; it emphasizes the diagnostic techniques that I have personally found to be most successful. Of central importance are the narratives, authentic case presentations that repeat the interchanges between me and my child patients; it is by recounting such stories that I believe the reader can best "feel his way" into the actual interview situations described.

Obviously, it would be difficult to try to set down rigid procedures for conducting interviews. It is easier and more accurate to demonstrate by example how particular problems of relating with children have been approached. The anecdotal-dialogue method adopted here has several advantages: first, it helps decrease the inevitable distortion that writing about interpersonal events produces—and any diagnostic interview with a child is above all an interpersonal event. Furthermore, it illustrates the importance of using language appropriate to the age of the child, it demonstrates the value of conducting an interview within a context appropriate to the situation, and it shows how empathy with the particular mood of the parents or the child can help bring a positive response.

The initial impetus that led me to undertake this book came from the residents training in general psychiatry at Rollman Psychiatric Institute in Cincinnati, Ohio. For the past six years I have taught seminars on the diagnostic process in child psychiatry at this particular training center. The outlines for these seminars formed the framework for the chapters in this book. Avid learners, the residents at Rollman's responded best, I felt, to a thoroughly clinical, anecdotal approach. What helped them most, in learning about evaluating children, was a show-and-tell methodology: I would conduct demonstration interviews with children and their families, and at other times I would tell numerous stories about the evaluation of other troubled children.

In this way the trainees could begin to project themselves into the role of interviewer and to perceive more clearly the nature of the diagnostic process. The aim is to help them overcome much of the natural anxiety of the beginning interviewer and also to bridge the inevitable gap between theory and practice. Accordingly, there are many clinical stories sprinkled throughout the book. In most cases, a story is used to illustrate a particular method or technique for evaluating children, then conclusions based on the clinical experience are stated. These should verbalize and therefore reinforce the reader's own conclusions reached after going through the story.

The focus of the writing is not on basic psychodynamics, although the varied forces that contribute to shaping children's behavior often emerge in the course of the case histories. In the process of evaluating children, interviewers obtain historical data and impressions of personal feelings from their young subjects and from their families that, when added up, lead to what Dr. Othilda Krug, my former training director in child psychiatry at the University of Cincinnati, often referred to as "psychodynamics plainly viewed—dynamics worth their salt are the ones that generally fall out in front of you on the table." The study of the psychodynamic forces affecting children is implicit in the diagnostic process, and a diagnostic evaluation, properly conducted, will often allow such forces to surface with the kind of common-sense clarity Dr. Krug referred to.

The book presupposes that trainees or mental health associates who are about to begin evaluating children have a thorough grounding in the normative facts of child development. Among the best sources of such data for our trainees have been the developmental section of Hale F. Shirley's book, *Pediatric Psychiatry*; the splendid *Group for the Advancement of Psychiatry Report No. 38*, "The Diagnostic Process in Child Psychiatry"; the Group for the Advancement of Psychiatry's monograph, *Normal Adolescence*; and Erik H. Erikson's book, *Childhood and Society*.[1] All of these provide a normative developmental yardstick against which the person evaluating children can measure his child patient. An excellent companion text that covers the area of psychopathology in children is the *Group for the Advancement of Psychiatry Report No. 62,*

1. Shirley, *Pediatric Psychiatry* (Cambridge: Harvard Univ. Press, 1963), 207–420. *Group for the Advancement of Psychiatry Report No. 38*, "The Diagnostic Process in Child Psychiatry" (New York, 1957). Committee on Adolescence, Group for the Advancement of Psychiatry, *Normal Adolescence* (New York: Scribners, 1968). Erikson, *Childhood and Society* (New York: Norton, 1963).

"Psychopathological Disorders in Childhood: Theoretical Considerations and a Proposed Classification."[2] This particular classification of children's psychopathology is the one used here throughout.

The book is structured along clinical, operational lines. Each chapter's heading and content follow the actual steps one can take in conducting a diagnostic evaluation of a child and his family. Thus there are chapters dealing with, in turn, considerations of the diagnostic process as a whole; parental inquiries initiating an evaluation; interview settings; meeting parents jointly in the initial interview; meeting the child in several diagnostic sessions; further individual interviews the evaluator may have with each parent; elective procedures that often facilitate the diagnostic study; and, finally, the follow-up conference with the parents that concludes the diagnostic evaluation of their child. At the end of the book is an extensive Appendix containing materials generally useful in the diagnostic study. The part that each item in the Appendix plays in the diagnostic process is emphasized in the text at the point where these materials are first introduced to the family and to the child himself during the evaluation.

The clinical work on which this book is based has depended upon the cooperation and support of literally hundreds of people. No acknowledgments can adequately express my appreciation of their help, including the clinical insights they have fostered.

First of all are those more than nine hundred families from the urban areas in and around Baltimore, Cincinnati, and Lexington and from the rural counties of central and eastern Kentucky who must remain unnamed—families with whom my colleagues and I were privileged to work and consult over the past fourteen years. They are wonderful, unforgettable families. Unnamed also, but equally important, are the local community leaders, school superintendents, teachers, and primary physicians and the staffs of various other service agencies with whom I discussed specific clinical and more general regional problems bearing on the evaluation of children they referred to me. I have drawn the stories for the book from the lives of these families I've known through the

2. New York, 1966.

years. The names of children and their families, as well as certain other identifying information, were of course altered to ensure confidentiality of the clinical information based on their lives.

Furthermore, I must underscore my debt to the earlier and continuing work of others in the area of evaluating children. Drs. Reginald Lourie and Othilda Krug, who were my training directors, their staffs, and the many others who have worked at evaluating children on a long-term basis have contributed much to my own growth and development as a person and as a career child psychiatrist. If in some ways my observations and suggestions recorded here are accurate and helpful, this service will constitute a small tribute to those who have taught me.

No words of mine can fully express the indebtedness I owe to editorial writer Thomas Parrish of Berea, Kentucky. His patient labors over this manuscript, and over the manuscript for my earlier book, *Appalachia's Children*,[3] are truly appreciated.

Once before, in 1970, while writing *Appalachia's Children*, I had occasion to express gratitude and apology to my wife Glyndon, son John, and daughter Mary, whose initial encouragement reinforced the suggestions of others that that book be written and who continued to provide support through the many months required for its completion. An event occurred while I was writing *Appalachia's Children* that perhaps serves to point up what can be one's overall approach to talking with children in evaluation interviews.

One evening, at the end of a week during which I had come home hurriedly from the clinic each day, bolted down my supper, and immediately secluded myself in the study (with instructions to my family not to interrupt me), our son John violated the injunction at one point. He knocked on the door about nine, apologized, and said he would just tiptoe over to the bookcase for a reference work. Swallowing some irritation, I wrote on, my back to John's fumbling about on the bookshelf. Finished, he crept out, closing the door softly behind him. About twenty minutes later I was startled to hear John's voice calling "Dad, are you there?" It came from one

---

3. *Appalachia's Children: The Challenge of Mental Health* (Lexington: Univ. Press of Kentucky, 1971).

of his walkie-talkies he had planted in the bookcase earlier. John was reestablishing contact with me, his absent father, by the only available avenue of communication that circumstances permitted that week! The action was effective; it got my attention in a way that broke us all up in laughter and led us to spend a brief period that evening as a reunited family.

Moreover, the event had an effect on me long after its initial impact on that particular evening. It pointed up a most important, perhaps even central, theme that guides my feelings toward, my thinking about, and my behavior in evaluating children: namely, that children have their own unique, inimitable ways of communicating their needs to others. How much this fact can aid us as interviewers with children! Now, instead of anxiously awaiting our first interviews with children, we can relax somewhat, confident that the youngsters we see will find a way to let us know how they are doing. Much of the burden of communicating is borne, then, by the child himself. His behavior tells us this, and it implies something more: our part, as evaluating grownups, is first and foremost to help the child relate with us. Once relationships are established, he will generally provide us with all the information he feels we need to know to assist him with his troubles. Our second task, to listen carefully to what the child says and to observe him carefully in his play, in his talk, and in his various moods, is made easier when the child has freed us to do so by taking much of the burden of communication on his own shoulders. Let us, therefore, as those called upon to evaluate children, keep to our part. We can be assured the children will generally do theirs.

Contents

Getting
to Know
the Troubled
Child

Chapter 1.

The Diagnostic Process: An Overview

People who work with children, or intend to do so, have a number of special traits in common; and, whatever their individual backgrounds, these are traits that stem from their own childhood days. The most important are a certain sensitivity to the feelings of children, an awareness of the psychological forces at work within families, a capacity to empathize with people, and a desire to help others. Perhaps we should add a liking for children—an indispensable quality for one who works with them. Those of us who possess such qualities, whether consciously or unconsciously, are frequently led in the direction of clinical work with children. However, anyone who actually enters the field rapidly becomes aware that receptivity to people is only the beginning of the job—we need to add refinement and methodology to our personal skills.

GENERAL CONSIDERATIONS

The diagnostic evaluation of a child might be defined as the process by which the evaluator, the parents, and the child himself investigate together the child's relative successes and failures in mastering certain tasks that confront all children as they move through the several stages of personality development. Such a definition depends on certain general principles of child development.

Field of Forces. The first of these, simply stated, is that children do not grow up in a vacuum. The children we see for evaluation are in a real sense not "all children." They cannot be understood apart from the historical, geographic, and socio-economic characteristics of the area in which they live. Thus to attain full knowledge of these children we have to acquire a great deal of information about the lives of their parents, their teachers, and the many other persons upon whom they are dependent. The well-rounded assessment of a child takes note not only of his own physical and psychological functioning but also of the entire field of forces within which he grows up, for his development is guided—or misguided—by the feelings, ideas, and behavior of other people.

Involving those who have influenced his environment is important for further reasons. Since the time interval between the child's birth and his referral for evaluation is a matter of years, not—as in adults—of decades, parental memories of the pregnancy and the postnatal period are usually sharp enough to supplement data we obtain from hospital charts and pediatric records. Similarly, the almost constant supervision required by the preschool child makes it possible to obtain detailed information about his day-to-day behavior from his parents. And teachers know the degree to which the school-age child learns, socializes with his peers, and conforms to the other demands of school. Unlike the adult, the child is gauged by persons whose professional responsibility it is to observe and evaluate him.[1] And even when the parents' views of the causes of the child's troubles are considered to be of questionable value, their reports concerning his birth, development, and current behavior and feelings may generally be considered reliable.

Complexity. The second of the general developmental issues that bear upon our evaluation of children is that the behavior of any person, child or adult, over his life span is complex beyond description; human behavior, we recognize, always has many causes. Under these circumstances the best we can do as evaluators (and I imply no disparagement) is to discern

1. Eli M. Bower, *Early Identification of Emotionally Handicapped Children in School* (Springfield: Charles C. Thomas, 1960). Dr. Bower, in this particular research study, found that both elementary school teachers and their students were only slightly less capable than an orthopsychiatric team of designating accurately those children in the schools surveyed who had mental health problems requiring treatment. See also Eli M. Bower, "Primary Prevention in a School Setting," in *Prevention of Mental Disorders in Children*, ed. Gerald Caplan (New York: Basic Books, 1961), 353-77.

developmental order through the diagnostic process with a family. Using the facts and feelings gathered from the child and from the other people concerned, we can see forces and factors that enable us to compare the early and later life relationships and functioning of the child. During the diagnostic process, we tease out, as it were, some crucial factors without expecting to uncover all of them. The evaluation of a child is, thus, the most accurate crosssectional view of his overall present functioning we are likely to get. Simultaneously, the evaluation takes into account the fact that the child is a developing person, growing up within a physical-psychological-social field of forces that, through its operation in the past and present, has much to do with shaping his behavior. This point is also made by the Committee on Child Psychiatry of the Group for the Advancement of Psychiatry in their report "The Diagnostic Process in Child Psychiatry":

> The diagnostic process, therefore, must include two essential areas of investigation, each with its special characteristics but each understood more fully in its reciprocal relationship with the other. These are (1) the child himself, his basic physical and intellectual endowment and the inner biological and psychological forces and behavior patterns or ego mechanisms which emerge in the development of his own individual identity, and (2) the environment and its social forces which influence the child as he matures. In the exploration of dynamic and psychogenetic factors, any unilateral approach precludes accurate diagnosis. The child, his family, and his society must be understood separately and in their interactions.[2]

DEVELOPMENTAL CONSIDERATIONS

Making a comprehensive evaluation, as previously defined, involves primarily an investigation of the child's relative successes and failures in mastering in orderly sequence certain universal tasks, and of the attendant anxieties that confront all children as they move through the several stages of personality development. An accurate assessment of a child depends, obviously, on the body of knowledge we have about normal

2. *Group for the Advancement of Psychiatry Report No. 38.*

personality growth. It is crucial that the findings we obtain during the diagnostic process be measured against the developmental norms for the successive stages of growth. Basic to this concept is the idea that normal personality patterns evolve out of interpersonal relationships. As a unique, distinct biosocial person, the child is always interacting with others, especially his family, during his early, formative years.

So it is that the frequency and severity of various psychopathological symptoms in any given population of adults and children appear to be markedly affected by social relationships and cultural values. Those who have a strong social-learning-theory orientation to child development, as I have, tend to view psychopathology in children as primarily involving learned behaviors, which are reinforced by environmental influences.[3]

The structure of adult society and of its smaller unit, the family, provides a context within which the growing child interprets his experience. It also influences the kind of mental "set" with which the child approaches new experiences. Viewed in this manner, family and regional cultural training patterns, which may vary from one family, one region, or one culture to another, are economical. The consistency with which they are set and maintained is important, of course. A training pattern allows the child—as it does any one of us—to be comfortable in his own environment. It facilitates the acquisition of the generally efficient behaviors we describe as socialization and acculturation.

Training Patterns. Although consistent family and regional training patterns result in appropriate, efficient behaviors in children within their cultural setting, the same training processes can also make it uncomfortable for an individual when

3. Joseph W. Eaton and Robert J. Weil, for example, feel that the data they gained from a mental health study of a Hutterite population fit this theory well; see *Culture and Mental Disorders: A Comparative Study of the Hutterites and Other Populations* (Glencoe, N. Y.: Free Press, 1955), 135. Adult patients in the Hutterite group had chiefly those neurotic symptoms which were socially acceptable in their culture. They took their tensions out on themselves by internalizing them as depression or psychophysiologic responses. Phobic and obsessive-compulsive reactions, which would violate strong cultural taboos, were rare. Within their highly structured social system, Hutterite individuals also were sufficiently sheltered and guided to make generalized anxiety reactions rare. However, adult Hutterites who moved from their structured communities to new locations frequently developed anxiety and phobic reactions to stress after a time. Their former coping defenses, previously applicable through group reinforcement, were no longer available to them in these new settings, and symptoms developed.

change is called for. A child who has been babied, for example, may adapt easily to an overprotective home environment during his preschool years. After starting school, he may become anxious on finding that his previously learned dependent behaviors run counter to the school's desire that he function more assertively and more autonomously.

Those who have worked with Southern Appalachian migrants in urban settings, to cite another example, are aware of this same kind of phenomenon, which may occur in one or more members of a family after changing their cultural location. The demand for new kinds of behavior conflicts strongly with the inflexible patterns already set. A family may be able to live in a marginally satisfactory way within the culture of origin for years, yet develop overt psychopathological symptoms after moving to a cultural setting that demands new behaviors.

Such points serve to remind us that the children we see are members not only of families but also of wider groups whose training patterns affect them a great deal. As evaluators, we need to be aware of these cultural patterns if we are to gain a fuller understanding of the child's own functioning and that of his family. In the Southern Appalachian region, for example, the training patterns, or models that families provide for their children's behavior, are relatively undiluted by social institutions outside the family. The close-knit, interdependent, extended family system is the only major social unit. It therefore holds a unique place as a child's training climate. And more often than not, the few social institutions available there outside the families have, up to now, served only to reinforce the established training patterns, which appear to have been remarkably consistent within the region through several generations. In my earlier book, *Appalachia's Children*, I outlined some of the most prominent among these practices, considering each one with reference to its implication for the mental health or mental disorder of the children we saw in field clinics. It was striking, indeed, to see the connections that exist between Southern Appalachian regional child development and the psychopathology of children from that area.[4]

The growing-up process in any region can be defined operationally as the acquisition of a particular set of facts and skills.

4. Pp. 18-22.

Its success is measured by the rapidity with which the child achieves the goals his environment sets for him. As already stated, these demands are extremely complex, and their details vary from one culture to the next. But in essence they are the same: the child is expected to master the basic abilities that his environment requires for biologic and social life. The following list includes the abilities needed in our culture and in most others:

1. Intellectual capacity.
2. Capacity for purposive and coordinated movement.
3. Degree of attainment of the orderly habits of eating and excretion, of regular cycles of sleep and wakefulness, and of a variety of self-help tasks.
4. Degree of attainment of understandable communication and social language.
5. Capacity for object relations with parents, other adults, siblings, and peers.
6. Degree of attainment of well-modulated expression of emotional reactions to the environment.
7. Nature of self-concept, self-awareness, and self-esteem.
8. Reality testing—this includes the child's perceptual capacities and other cognitive functions.
9. Nature of superego operations (conscience and ego-ideal) —the degree of the child's acceptance of prohibitions and sanctions, prevailing customs, and ideas of decency.
10. Degree of attainment of an orderly pursuit of knowledge and education.
11. Adaptive or integrative capacity—including capacity for meeting and mastering tasks; capacity for understanding and synthesizing the thoughts and feelings connected with events; the capacity for self-observation; the capacity to store tension, which includes the level of frustration tolerance, the level of inner controls on impulses, and the ability to delay gratification; the capacity to sublimate feelings; and the capacity to remember and to recall events.
12. Current level of psychosocial development—with reference to the various stages of development, including an assessment of fixations, regressions, or developmental deviations.
13. Basic personality structure (basic life-style).

14. Areas of psychological conflict—and whether the conflicts in the child are largely internal or external or both.
15. Predominant defensive and adaptive capacities (ego defense mechanisms).
16. Degree of impairment in capacity for physical development, play, learning, or socialization.
17. An assessment of the degree to which all of these abilities, or ego functions, have been integrated into behavior in the child that is well balanced between the family's and the community's expectations for him and his own self-interest.

The above list of children's ego functions was adapted from a very similar one contained in the *Group for the Advancement of Psychiatry Report No. 62*, "Psychopathological Disorders in Childhood: Theoretical Considerations and a Proposed Classification," and from the comments made by Gilbert H. Glaser, Jonathan Pincus, and Sally A. Provence in the book *Modern Psychiatric Treatment*.[5] This list forms a helpful guide for the collection of data during the diagnostic process. It is also valuable as a shorthand way of thinking through and writing up the diagnostic evaluation of the child.

PSYCHOPATHOLOGICAL CONSIDERATIONS

The family and the community regard "disorder" in a child as that state in which he complies poorly or not at all with some or all of their training demands. "Pathology" is the manner in which this noncompliance becomes manifest. The younger the child, the less his family and community usually expect of him, and the less likely his unusual behavior is to be considered evidence of a disorder. The older he gets, the more is expected of him, and, accordingly, the wider is the variety of disorders to which he can be subject. What the family and the community expect of a given child reflects their experience with other children of the same age in the community. Every child as he grows up is constantly

5. "Psychiatric Illness in Childhood," in *Modern Psychiatric Treatment*, eds. Thomas P. Detre and Henry G. Jarecki (Philadelphia: Lippincott, 1971).

measured against his peers. His relative successes or failures in defining, meeting, and mastering various tasks are constantly compared with the progress made by other children. But these publicly derived peer norms cannot be applied too rigidly. Not only does the overall rate of development vary widely among children, but the rate of growth for different skills in a particular child may be quite uneven.

Because each child's maturation depends on the orderly acquisition of skills and each new skill becomes a part of the foundation for the next, even a mild slowing or unevenness in development can sometimes give the appearance of gross abnormality. The identification of abnormal behavior in a child is further complicated because behavior that is considered pathologic at one age may be common or even universal at another. For example, head-banging, thumbsucking, and rocking are very common in infants and toddlers. Crying spells, temper tantrums, bedwetting, nightmares, hyperactivity, dialogues with imaginary playmates, and refusing to eat, to go to bed, to greet visitors, or to be separated from the parents are among the many kinds of behavior that are regarded as normal in the child up to the age of four or five but would be indicative of a disorder in an older child. On the other hand, the overt expression of sexual interest is regarded as normal after puberty but abnormal before that age.

Peer Norms. Nonetheless, peer norms for the various ego functions are still the best yardsticks against which we, as evaluators, measure children. They are also the guides used by others. When a child is referred to us, he has been designated as having emotional or learning problems by other persons in his cultural setting—parents, teachers, physician, court or other agency, or public health nurse. This initial labeling of a child as maladjusted in some way is essentially a culture-based definition based on peer norms for various behaviors.

The same peer-norm yardstick by which to measure psychopathology in children guided the Committee on Child Psychiatry of the Group for the Advancement of Psychiatry as they recently recommended and outlined a new diagnostic nomenclature for psychopathological disorders of children. I have found this classification very useful in my own clinical work because it represents the most recent national consensus of child psychiatrists and others, and the descriptions of the various categories of disorder are clear and accurate. Generally, it is relatively easy to match the child one has evaluated with one of these descriptions. I also feel that presenting my clinical material according to this proposed national classification standard enhances communication with other clinicians and researchers.[6]

SUMMARY OF THE DIAGNOSTIC PROCESS

The person who evaluates a child brings to the diagnostic process his knowledge of human behavior, gained from the rich variety of his own experiences throughout life and from his professional training. He sees individual personality development as a continuum from infancy through childhood (with its toddler, preschool, and middle childhood periods) and adolescence to adulthood. He will also be familiar with the psychodynamics operating in the lives of children and their families and the psychopathology of children. He is aware, too, of the importance of cultural training patterns in child development, and thus he is alert to the ways in which specific patterns have contributed to the life of the child before him. He comes with a desire to understand the child and his family, to clarify situations, and to assist parents in redirecting certain aspects of their child's growth. He is sensitive to the feelings of others and, very probably, likes children. All of this is his preparation, and by being prepared he is in a reasonable position to evaluate a child.

To this background the evaluator adds his understanding that the diagnostic study itself is a dynamic process offering new relationships and potentially valuable experiences to the child and his parents as they are helped to face their problems together. He realizes that the study is based on a sound knowledge of both normal and pathological development and function

6. The classification of children's psychopathology referred to is found throughout the *Group for the Advancement of Psychiatry Report No. 62.*

and on an awareness of the continuous interaction of all the psychobiological and psychosocial forces. This understanding demands a multifaceted approach. No unilateral study can effectively reveal the crosscurrents and significant forces in a total family situation. Sufficient historical data about physical, psychological, and social factors are needed. There must be an adequate evaluation of the child's current levels of physical and psychological functioning and valid appraisals of his native physical equipment and his intellectual endowment.

The evaluator must also be aware that the diagnostic process frequently needs to be a collaborative one, requiring the specialized methods of several professional disciplines to investigate the various diagnostic areas. Some settings, like psychiatric clinics for children, are staffed and structured on this basic assumption. Personnel from each of the various medical and nonmedical specialties may be there under one roof to add knowledge from each of their areas to the comprehensive study of the child. In many other settings, however, some—or even most—of the specialties that may be needed to complete the thorough case review indicated for a particular child are lacking. Nor does every troubled child referred for evaluation require, in the words of one of my former trainees, "the million-dollar workup." That important determination is made by the person, of whatever basic professional discipline, who assumes primary responsibility for the evaluation of the child. It is incumbent upon him, as he begins to work with the child and the family, to determine whether and in what area the further diagnostic skills and methods of a collaborator are called for. If the need exists, he can arrange for a physical or neurological evaluation of the child, clinical psychological testing, a speech and hearing assessment, a thorough review by another diagnostic clinic if mental retardation is suspected, and so on. Sometimes he must reach beyond his own office, clinic, or agency, or even his own community, to obtain the diagnostic services of one of these other specialists. This takes time, diligence, and patience, and it requires the evaluator to assume the leadership and direction of the overall diagnostic study. The responsibility for synthesizing the various diagnostic data into a comprehensive diagnosis of the child in his environment is one of our greatest challenges.

The separate diagnostic areas involved in the evaluation of a child, the specific procedures and techniques that enable us to investigate each of these areas, and the ways in which each area contributes to the total diagnostic formulation are considered in detail in the next chapters. And, very importantly, there will also be some discussion of appropriate ways to feed back information to the child and family with whom we are working, as the diagnostic process continues, so that all of us are truly tackling the job together.

In the next chapter we meet the family where the evaluator first meets them—over the telephone, as someone calls to seek help for a troubled child.

Chapter 2.

Meeting the Family:
The Inquiry

About three o'clock one October afternoon, the telephone rang in my office. The caller identified herself as Alice Russell. Obviously distraught, she immediately began to talk about the problems she and her husband were having with their son Charlie. "Tom and I are so upset, and you've just got to help us, Dr. Looff! We were both called to the school this morning for a conference with Charlie's teacher—and they're about ready to throw him out of class. He's acting up again—disrupting the group and hitting the other kids, and then he's not completing his work. And that's only half of it—he's been attacking his sister with scissors again." She paused for breath, at which point I said, "Mrs. Russell, I can hear that you're pretty anxious about Charlie. And I need to hear some more about what bothers you about him. But I have someone in the office with me right now. So I wonder, Mrs. Russell, if I could call you back at the end of this hour, when I'm free to talk." Mrs. Russell sputtered: "Oh, I'm so sorry! I should have guessed you'd be busy. I'm so upset—you're right—and I just rattled on there. Of course, please call me back. I'm not going anywhere. I'll be here." She then gave me her home telephone number and hung up.

As I turned away from the telephone, I had several distinct impressions. It was abundantly clear that Alice Russell was upset over the problems her young son was having in school. Furthermore, she was concerned about the attack Charlie had made on his sister. In that first moment of inquiry, there was evidence that the boy was having problems both at school and at home. But Alice Russell had done more than talk about her son's problems. She had also revealed herself to be capable of looking at her feelings when I had reflected her anxiety back to her. She had agreed that what she was feeling was anxiety. Mrs. Russell therefore gave me the impression that she was capable of *consensual validation* of her feelings in a given situation.[1] Furthermore, she had clearly stated her observation that the force of her feelings had led her to plunge on without asking whether I was free to talk with her. In this way she had indicated both that social amenities were probably important to her and that, even in the face of her anxiety, she was not crippled by it but retained the capacity for accurate self-observation. And, finally, she had led me to believe that she could work cooperatively with me around problems the boy and the family were having.

Mrs. Russell's call that afternoon was fairly typical of an inquiry for help with a troubled child. Her call highlighted the specific differences between inquiries made by adults—as in adult psychiatry—and those made in behalf of children. The adult patient usually presents himself for evaluation because of symptoms from which he seeks relief. With the exception of the psychotic patient or the individual who is referred by an authoritative agency such as a court, the adult seeks help from the evaluator voluntarily, although often reluctantly. The young child or adolescent, on the other hand, seldom if ever seeks help for himself but is brought to the evaluator by his parents or other adults responsible for his care. Often they do so out of their own concern about the child's adjustment, but frequently such a move has been recommended or even ordered by persons or agencies in a position to do so. In the case of the Russells, the recommendation of the school that the parents seek psychiatric aid for Charlie apparently reinforced their already present concerns about the boy's home adjustment. The school's report of Charlie's maladjustment had upset them. But obviously it did not make them defensive about, or resistive to, the need to inquire about psychiatric services for the boy. That point was implicit, too, in Mrs. Russell's initial call.

Her call pointed up another important aspect of the referral-inquiry part of the diagnostic process. In most cases

1. "Consensual validation" is a term used frequently by Harry Stack Sullivan, a psychiatrist, to describe the mutual process of clarification of historical events and attendant feelings engaged in by the interviewer and the patient in a diagnostic study. See Harry S. Sullivan, *The Interpersonal Theory of Psychiatry* (New York: Norton, 1953), 28-29.

of this type, the most significant complaints about the troubled child are those given initially and spontaneously. Sometimes these complaints do not concur precisely with those of the teacher or community agency worker who has stimulated the application. Parents may view their child's behavior in a different manner from that of the teacher or others, perhaps because they deny the existence of problems in their child and thereby significantly distort their view of him. But sometimes the child's behavior at school is truly different from his behavior at home. In the initial call from Mrs. Russell, however, there was a strong hint that she saw the same problems in Charlie as his teacher did; this agreement between their views of Charlie's behavior was significant.

TYPES OF REFERRALS

In a *school* referral of a child for evaluation, the chief concern is apt to be the child's academic achievement or social adjustment. School personnel are usually concerned particularly over underachieving, aggressive, impulsive, or poorly socialized children. More and more, however, teachers are becoming aware of the needs of shy, withdrawn, and fearful children as well. Often they are also able to spot the learning problems in younger school-age children that suggest specific learning disabilities. School referrals are becoming increasingly sophisticated and accurate as individual teachers, from their practical experience and from training in child development and psychopathology in children, are made aware of the entire range of problems troubled children may have.

In a *court* referral, the emphasis will be on symptomatic delinquent behavior. For example, parents may have filed an out-of-control, incorrigibility petition asking a juvenile court to assume custody of their adolescent boy or girl, who may be running away, engaging in promiscuous sexual activity, or involved in drug abuse. In planning for the adolescent, the court may request an evaluation by community clinic personnel or by a consultant in private practice. Some juvenile courts in large urban areas have their own multidisciplinary staffs for evaluations. Like the courts, many city, regional, and state public assistance and child welfare agencies are concerned with needy, dependent, impulsive, poorly socialized children. It is these behaviors that lead them to make referrals for evaluation and planning on behalf of the child. Because most of these agencies do not have personnel beyond their own social work staffs, they must turn outside for this type of assistance.

In the *medical* referral of a child, a primary physician—whether he is a generalist, a pediatrician, or another medical specialist— will put more emphasis on specific neurotic or psychotic symptomatology, psychosomatic disorders, or developmental deviations. Many requests from primary physicians are for consultations on hospitalized children. Referrals also may be suggested to parents by physicians who see the children in their private office or clinic practices.

Thus the source of referral of a troubled child may be the parents themselves, the school, the court, the social agency, or the pediatrician or other physician. Inquiries may come in from parents acting on their own concerns about their child, from parents who have been encouraged to seek referral by someone else, or from other persons who have some responsibility for the child's development and training.

The Evaluator's Tasks. Whenever someone other than the child's parents calls him directly, the evaluator has several crucial tasks: (1) He must listen carefully to the observations that are made about the child's behavior. As a means both of getting these observational data down accurately and of reinforcing the positive effort the caller is making in behalf of the child, I tell him or her, early in the call, that I am making verbatim notes of the conversation. This indicates, more than anything else I could say over the telephone, that I'm listening carefully and also that I place great importance on the data I'm receiving. Again, as with the inquiries parents make directly, the evaluator attaches particular significance to those observations about the child given initially and spontaneously by the teacher or physician. After getting this first information, the evaluator can then learn what else the caller may know about the child's functioning by asking questions about specific areas of behavior the caller may not have mentioned. Much additional and invaluable information may be gained in this manner. And, again, the referring person feels that his opinions count with the evaluator. This type of approach, I have found, helps one develop and maintain good working relationships with teachers, physicians, and others who may be referring sources.

(2) Toward the end of a direct call from a referring teacher or physician, the evaluator must indicate that he is now aware of the caller's concerns from what has been said, and that from this information he agrees (if this is indeed the case) that further review of the child is warranted. He then either indicates his own readiness to conduct the evaluation or, if necessary, suggests another person or agency.

(3) At this point the evaluator should find out whether the person calling has discussed his feelings with the family. This step is a truly important one. It can help ensure that the parents will in due course be accessible for truly collaborative work with the evaluator. Teachers and physicians who understand this generally agree, in response to the evaluator's request, to get in touch with the parents, either in person or by telephone, to talk over the child's problems. They attempt to reflect the parents' own anxiety in a manner that will help them see the need for an evaluation, mentioning that these concerns have been discussed with the evaluator and suggesting that the parents call him directly. This route of referral is a truly collaborative one. But some referral sources do not understand this process. The evaluator must help such callers see that any evaluation will be essentially ineffectual, so far as working well with the family is concerned, if parents are simply told by the referring doctor or teacher to call for evaluation appointments without further explanation. They deserve a frank personal discussion of the need for the review; if it is not given, they may well refuse to cooperate fully later. Thus the future evaluator can serve as an educator for the most appropriate referral process. Even so, some callers may still have great difficulty in working supportively with families in the ways indicated here. As evaluators of these families, then, we frequently do inherit the guardedness and the resistances to the diagnostic process itself that are symptomatic of this lapse in procedure.

(4) At the very end of the call the evaluator indicates clearly that he will be in touch with the referring person, generally by telephone, at the end of the diagnostic study, in order to share his findings and to discuss future treatment goals and

plans, an important aspect of which includes the mutually agreed-upon roles the teacher, the family physician, and the evaluator will play. This commitment to the referring person is a very important one indeed for the future collaborative work with the troubled child. The process of mutually defining each person's role in a treatment plan for a child will come up again in this book, when treatment planning at the end of an evaluation is discussed in much fuller detail. But the concept is always introduced by the evaluator at the time of inquiry from a referring person. And, again, this kind of commitment facilitates the development and maintenance of good working relationships with people who not only refer children but also have an important part to play in the children's further growth and development.

CONDUCT OF THE INQUIRY

Regardless of the source or manner of the referral, the areas of investigation that begin at the time of the parents' inquiry are:

(1) a historical résumé of their child's problems—an overview of what concerns them most about him;

(2) what feelings are currently stirred up in parents as a result of the child's behavior;

(3) what attitudes and feelings parents have toward obtaining help from the evaluator; and

(4) closely allied with (3), a beginning hint of what the parents expect from the evaluation—what it is they would like the evaluator to do for them and their child.

As one former trainee paraphrased it: "It boils down, at the time of inquiry, to finding out who is complaining, about what, and what it is they want of you."

Alice Russell, when I had fifteen minutes' time in which to call her back, spoke spontaneously to these four points as she enlarged upon her earlier telephone inquiry: "Dr. Looff, Charlie's so active. He runs all over the place, and just won't mind me at all. My husband has an easier time controlling him, and that makes me feel even worse. I feel I ought to be doing something more to control Charlie, but I'm just not sure what it is.

Tom tells me to stand up to him, but when I try Charlie just grins, or gets angry and runs away. I'm left completely frustrated and angry, and sooner or later I blow my stack and spank him. Then I feel guilty—I don't like to lose control of my temper. But I can't help it—Charlie stirs me up so!''

She went on to say that the discipline problem was nothing new but had existed for seven years—in fact, ever since Charlie was born. "Sounds funny, I know, but that's a fact. Tom says it's all my fault, not being firm enough with Charlie all along. But I've been so confused about how to handle him for so long. And I've got such different kinds of advice. Tom's either not home, so it's left up to me, or he blames me for being such a poor disciplinarian when he is home. And then our pediatrician has told me all along that Charlie will grow out of this. He says I worry too much. Actually, Dr. Thompson really isn't in favor of an evaluation." But, Mrs. Russell said, Charlie had been getting so impatient with his four-year-old sister, Elizabeth, that she was sure something was wrong. And even her husband was beginning to agree.

And now, she said, "the school says there's something wrong there, too. Charlie is destructive of papers and things, often hits the other children without warning, won't pay attention in class, and doesn't finish any of his papers. Mrs. Snyder, his teacher, says he won't make it through the year if this keeps up. In fact, they told Tom and me in the conference at the school this morning that Charlie needs a psychological evaluation. They said that if we don't do this, and get help for Charlie, they will have to suspend him from school, perhaps indefinitely. But he is such a friendly and likable boy at other times. He's bright, too, I can tell that."

As Mrs. Russell paused, I had an opportunity to restate the child's problems and the many feelings in response to them that she had given me. This act of reflecting their statements about problems and associated feelings reinforces the parents' beginning awareness of the difficulties their child is having. By such reflection they feel not only that they are listened to but also that the statements and feelings are themselves important to them and to the evaluator. Such reflection may also suggest to them, as the evaluation proceeds, that other problem-oriented statements and associated feelings they can share may be similarly crucial in understanding the child and the family.

Mrs. Russell responded to my reflection by indicating that I had understood her correctly. At this point, I asked her what it was she hoped to gain from me—what it was she wanted me to do. This she indicated clearly: "Actually, I know you can't give Charlie a pill or something and clear this up overnight. But maybe you can tell us why he does these things. I've wondered if maybe he's brain-damaged. Tom pooh-poohs that idea. But it's stuck in my mind. I asked Mrs. Snyder that, but she says she doesn't know much about brain-damaged children. Dr. Thompson, when I asked him about it, said he didn't think so. He did put Charlie on Ritalin two weeks ago, though, but it only made him groggy, so I discontinued it. Do you think he may be brain-damaged? Or is it emotional problems, as Mrs. Snyder thinks it is? I'm just not sure."

Here I reflected to Mrs. Russell that it seemed to me that she was pointing up the very real need for a complete differential diagnostic evaluation of her son. She agreed with me, and indicated further that Tom was ready now "to go along with whatever you need to do to find out what is the matter with Charlie."

I then asked Mrs. Russell how she had happened to call me for help with her son. That answer, too, was explicit: "Mrs. Snyder suggested your name in the conference this morning. On the way home, Tom said he didn't make enough, he thought, on his salary to pay for private care—but he trusted Mrs. Snyder's judgment. Tom's so definite about things. He wants you to see Charlie even though he feels a little embarrassed coming to you, because he likes to pay his bills on time. He told me to ask you if you would see Charlie, if we could pay you back over a long time from our budget." I indicated to Mrs. Russell that I was pleased that, in spite of conflicting feelings, her husband felt free to have her call me for the evaluation. And I told her we could later work out a fee and payment schedule.

The Six-Interview Format. Then I outlined for Mrs. Russell the format I use for a differential diagnostic evaluation of a child—the minimum number and type of diagnostic interviews we would probably need to schedule in order to complete an evaluation of Charlie.

(1) I like to meet just with parents in an initial *joint interview* focused on getting full information about the history

and current setting of the apparent problems in the child and their feelings about these problems.

(2) and (3) This initial interview is followed by *two separate interviews with the child alone*, in order that I may determine his own functioning in several areas.

(4) and (5) During this same time, but entirely separate from the interviews with the child, I have an *individual interview with the father* and *one with the mother*, each interview focused on my learning more about the personal functioning and social background of each of them—on my getting to know the parents better as people.

(6) Then, at the end of the evaluation, the parents and I meet in a *second joint interview*, to pool our emerging thoughts and feelings, to talk over the child as we all now see him, and to plan toward whatever steps might be indicated for his further care.

Mrs. Russell liked the thoroughness implicit in this six-interview evaluation format and agreed that we should work along this plan. She understood from what I said that this six-interview format was designed to be a kind of baseline for the differential diagnostic process and that, depending on the data emerging during the diagnostic study, we might need to schedule Charlie for an examination by a consulting neurologist, or a psychological evaluation, or perhaps other tests.

At this point I asked whether the boy had ever had previous psychiatric care of any kind. She indicated that they had taken him to a local child guidance clinic two years earlier for tests to obtain an estimate of his intellectual functioning, as required for entrance into a private kindergarten. I asked Mrs. Russell if she would be willing to ask this clinic to send me a copy of the results and interpretations of those tests. She indicated her willingness to do so. We closed our fifteen-minute telephone conversation by scheduling the initial, joint interview with Tom and herself to launch the diagnostic study.

From what Mrs. Russell had said about Charlie's problems, and from her own feelings and those of her husband, it was clear that I could anticipate meeting a couple who were in some disagreement but remained cooperative and sensitive—a couple who would probably be able during our later meetings to discuss a range of matters crucial to their son's problems, and would be capable of putting their feelings into words quite well. Hers was probably the most gratifying type of inquiry one can receive as an evaluator of children—and, happily, it is not uncommon.

In addition, Mrs. Russell's story serves as an example of the type of inquiry that generally leads the evaluator to plan a thorough diagnostic study. Chronic problems presented by children demand this long, hard look at the various biosocial and psychological contexts within which these behaviors occur. The six-interview format outlined here as a model for a thorough evaluation of a child is one I have found very useful in my own clincial work.

This type of plan can be used in both clinic and private-practice settings. Furthermore, it lends itself to the collaborative study of a particular child and his family. In clinics, for example, the psychiatrist or psychologist or psychiatric nurse or mental health associate—the evaluator of the child—may have a psychiatric social worker or another mental health associate on the staff to assist him. In that event, the social worker or mental health associate is the one who interviews the parents in the initial, joint session and in their separate sessions, whereas the primary evaluator of the child reserves his time for meeting solely with the child himself. As the diagnostic study proceeds, the child's evaluator and the social worker or mental health associate meet frequently to exchange emerging data, in order that they may remain properly in context. This way of working together is fairly typical for psychiatrists, social workers, psychologists, psychiatric nurses, mental health associates, and others in clinic settings. If he is in private practice, however, the evaluator may not have other staff working with him. The six-interview format then becomes a family study, in which the evaluator has the responsibility for conducting all of the interviews with the parents and their child.

Short-term Interviews. The above format cannot, however, be rigidly applied to all families. It is obvious that not all troubled children require the type of diagnostic study outlined here for the Russells. For example, some parents are concerned about very specific behaviors in their children, an outline of which at the time of their telephone inquiry clearly suggests to the evaluator that the child is generally functioning well except

in the one area being described by the caller. The evaluator
can validate his conclusion by asking the caller whether he is
"getting the correct picture of things from what you've been
saying." If the inquiring parent agrees, he and the evaluator
are then in a position to plan relatively short-term diagnostic-
treatment interviews for the family, having as their primary
goal the understanding of the stressful factors causing the problem behavior in the child and planning toward the alleviation
of these stresses.

An example of an inquiry from which I concluded that the
longer diagnostic study plan would be inappropriate is a call
I received one morning from Mrs. Evelyn Shugars concerning
her four-year-old son Chester: "Dr. Looff, my husband and I
are so upset with Chester—he just won't let me out of his sight.
It's like he's tied to my apron strings. Actually, he's not so
bad around the house, but when you try to get him to do
something on his own he balks like a mule! Why, just the other
day I had to drag him to our doctor's to get his Head Start
physical. Chester set his brakes and just wouldn't budge out
of the house!" Mrs. Shugars said she had bribed him to get
him to go, but once at the doctor's office Chester—"that big
baby"—had pitched "a real red fit right there in the waiting
room" and refused to leave her. "I sure was mad at him then,
I can tell you! The idea, not leaving me to go with the nurse!
It's so hard, though. Whenever I holler, like the other day, he
blubbers and says I don't love him anymore. That gets to me
—tears me all up inside. And then I give up and take him home"
—which she had done on this occasion. She made it plain that
she and her husband Frank, who were both in their forties,
loved Chester very much, saying that they had in fact tried for
twelve years to become parents. "And Dr. Becknell told me
the other day Chester's a good boy, Dr. Looff, and he is. But
he's just too tied to my apron strings. I really don't want that.
Frank and I want to come see you to find out what we're doing wrong with Chester. Maybe you can help us set him straight."

Mrs. Shugars's inquiry was fairly typical of the calls I receive
about overly dependent preschool children from close-knit
families in rural Kentucky. These children function generally
quite well except in the area of being able to separate from
their parents sufficiently to meet and master tasks on their
own. Typically, the parents of these children, whom I call

apron-string children, are, for a variety of reasons, overprotective and "infantilizing."[2] In effect, they train their children to be, as Evelyn described Chester, "big babies." I've learned that a relatively few diagnostic-treatment interviews focused on their mutual relationships with their preschool child often help these parents redirect their training efforts. That being so, I plan on short-term treatment interviews from the outset; this is discussed with the parents at the time of their initial inquiry. If, however, my first actual meeting with the parents uncovers data suggesting problems of greater depth and scope than the one described in their inquiry, then I tell the parents so, and we shift into the regular, longer diagnostic study.

Thus, the plan for the future diagnostic study—two types of which have been outlined here—takes its shape from the inquiry itself. That is true as well for families experiencing some sort of emotional crisis. If the parent who calls indicates that the problem concerns a school-phobic reaction, a suicidal attempt, or acutely antisocial and self-destructive behavior like fire-setting, stealing, drug abuse, sexual promiscuity, or running away from home, I treat it as an emergency situation. Accordingly, I plan that the first interview—set that day, if possible, or certainly no later than the next—include both parents and the child in joint session. They are put together onstage, as it were, to reveal ideas, feelings, and ways of relating together. This step is essential for possible crisis resolution, for planning for short-term management procedures, and for outlining further diagnostic-treatment sessions.

SUMMARY

Children do not come on their own for an evaluation of their troubled thoughts, feelings, and ways of behaving. Complaints about them are usually made by a parent or some other adult to whom the child's behavior presents a problem. These complaints generally come in the form of telephone inquiries. The most significant complaints are those given initially and spontaneously, even though they may not always concur precisely

---

2. David H. Looff, "The Apron-String Child," in *Feelings, 13* (Columbus, Ohio: Ross Laboratories), No. 3, May 1971.

with those suggested by the community resource person who may have stimulated the application. Regardless of the manner or source of the referral of a particular child, the evaluator gains from the inquiring parent impressions in four important areas: (1) a historical résumé of the child's problems—an overview of what concerns the parents most about the child; (2) what feelings are currently stirred up in parents as a result of the child's behavior; (3) what attitudes and feelings parents have toward obtaining help from the evaluator, and, closely allied with this, (4) a beginning hint of what it is the parents expect from the evaluator—what it is they would like him to do for them and their child.

With these four points in mind, the evaluator guides the inquiry. After he and the caller have reached mutual understanding on these matters, the plan for the diagnostic study can be shaped. Three types of diagnostic plans, all of which took their shape from parental inquiries, were outlined in this chapter.

The first, applicable to the Russell family, is used when there is a need for a thorough diagnostic study of a child with chronic learning and behavior problems. A six-interview format was outlined for this type of family study.

The second, applicable to the Shugars family, was given as an example of a study plan for a family having concerns about relatively selective, focused behaviors in an otherwise well-functioning child that seem amenable to short-term diagnostic-treatment interviews.

The third plan given was that applicable to a situation of family emotional crisis, where prompt, joint, entire-family interviews are imperative from the outset.

We meet the Russells and the Shugarses and families in crisis again when, in later chapters, the specific methods and procedures the evaluator can use in guiding the diagnostic study are reviewed in detail. But before the first face-to-face interviews, the evaluator must give consideration, also shaped by the inquiry, to the setting in which he will meet the family and the child. What works well in one situation may not be adequate in another. The next chapter takes up this important question.

Chapter 3.
Interview Settings

One day the Central Psychiatric Clinic at Cincinnati General Hospital registered Timothy Sizemore, a thin, watery-eyed farm lad who was dragged into the clinic by his angry mother. She had brought Tim, she told Mrs. Arletta Graves, the psychiatric social worker, to "have psychiatry done on him!" Her words epitomized her relationship with the boy. As the mother spat out her annoyance over Tim's severe stuttering, lifelong stubbornness, and fecal soiling, Mrs. Graves got an image of Tim as a toothpaste tube that his mother squeezed repeatedly in an attempt to produce something at both ends. It seemed quite clear from what she said explicitly and the feelings she revealed that Mrs. Sizemore hated men. She expressed this, I later saw, in such ways as constantly haranguing her husband, promptly selling the male foals dropped by the family's quarter horse mares, and repeatedly criticizing Tim and battling to control his functions.

No wonder, then, that Tim was so painfully shy that first afternoon with me, alone in the interview room at the clinic. I attempted to talk with him while Mrs. Graves interviewed his mother. Obviously anxious, Tim managed to squeak out only a few stuttered words that hour. He sat huddled miserably in a chair, his torn, ragged coat clutched over his chest as though he were wrapping himself away from a tormenting world. The inward pain I felt on seeing him thus must have been evident to the boy; my feelings tend to show. He smiled wanly at me, in what I took to be his way of showing me that he felt I understood his misery. I put our feelings into words, but Tim's shyness intervened, and he could say very little. But he listened intently as I described part of my own background as a farm boy from western Washington. That first interview ended on two shared points: Both Tim and I understood that he was feeling miserable, and we had established our mutual farm backgrounds. However, Tim was still too anxious to relate very much with me and to attempt to talk. This was hardly surprising. My newness, the frightening strangeness of the office set off in a hospital clinic (Tim rarely left his family's farm except to attend a local school), and the experience of being dragged in to "have psychiatry done on him" must have combined to make Tim feel so frightened and so inhibited.

Beyond these points, I could obviously draw no conclusions about Tim's functioning as a person. And it was obvious that I would have to see him further in a setting more familiar to him if both his problems and any strengths he might possess were to be properly assessed. I did not want to subject him to the total strangeness of the clinic office setting, on top of the hospital experience. I would therefore need to see him at his home, and in the immediate future.[1]

THE HOME SETTING

On a clear, snappy Saturday morning in early November I visited the Sizemore family's small farm, which was spread out on the top and over the sides of a long ridge in the southwest Ohio hill country bordering the Ohio River. Although still so painfully shy he avoided my face and hand in greeting and scuffed at the gravel in the yard with his shoes, Tim gave a weak smile. He seemed in this way to indicate that he was glad I had come. I told Tim that I would be very pleased to see his favorite haunts with him, and that maybe we could talk together as we went. We explored the house initially, because that was where Mrs. Sizemore told us we should go first. There, in the basement, in a small unheated room off the main cellar, Tim had a cot. The room was dimly lighted by a small, broken window up near the ceiling. Tim stuttered as he told me his fright over finding a black snake in his room one morning when he awoke. Evidently it had crawled in through the hole in the window. However, all was not pain there. Tim grinned shyly as he showed me the two pictures of farms he had cut out from old magazines and pinned to the wall above

1. Obtaining diagnostic material in the home setting of the child represents an adaptation of Erikson's anthropological field observational techniques. See Erikson, *Childhood and Society*, 54-56, 109-86.

his cot. Upstairs, we saw the three attractively decorated bedrooms belonging to his parents and his two younger sisters.

Then Tim and I went outside and walked the ridge and the woodlot, stirred up the muddy edge of the duck pond, admired the horses, and settled finally on the hood of one of several old cars relegated to a rusting junk pile on the edge of the woods. There Tim talked. Haltingly at first, but then in a rush of pained, stuttered words, he poured out his hope that someday he would be a "bachelor man" who worked on cars as a mechanic in their local town during the daytime, returning to his own farm in the evenings. "I'll have boy horses, too, and no one will ever yell at me again."

How clear it had all become! There in the familiar setting of his farm Tim could gradually thaw out to relate and talk with me. I learned that, although painfully shy, Tim could relate well and warmly, and that he possessed hopes that would be tapped in our future interviews to offset his doubts about himself. I had met Tim and his family onstage at their home. Their psychodynamics were poignantly clear in that setting. But the farm that morning had clearly provided more than a setting in which I obtained first-rate diagnostic material. It had, through its familiarity, brought pleasure both to Tim and to me, thereby enabling our relationship to deepen sufficiently to permit us to move on, not only to talk about Tim's worries and hopes there, but also to gain his agreement to holding our future talks in my office. Once he could accept me on his own ground, Tim could accept me anywhere. So armed, we could then get on with the task of finding out how he could meet many of his own needs himself—the work of future treatment interviews.

The conclusion I drew from this experience with Tim was that sometimes the setting of the interview with the child must be different from our customary one, or adapted to fit the child's functioning at the moment. The old Red Cross adage of "splint them where they lie" would seem to apply here. Frequently we as mental health professionals speculate about the transference factors or defensive resistances that make it difficult for the troubled child or his family to meet the interviewer in his accustomed office setting. We seem to be trying to fit the child into our setting. The practical point, however, is that some very fearful, very disturbed, or very shy children are scared out of their wits by an office setting that is familiar only to the interviewer. It takes only one interview of this type to convince the interviewer that some of these frightened children cannot be helped to share their troubled feelings in his office. In such a case, he is pointedly directed to shift his future interviews with the child to the familiar setting of the child's home. Often this shift of locale need involve only one home visit; sometimes several will be required. The goal is to enable the child to relate fairly well with the interviewer and to begin to tell of his hopes and fears. In these instances, as with Tim, the setting is determined by the child's needs.

THE HOSPITAL SETTING

There are, however, a number of circumstances in which the interviewer has no choice concerning the meeting place. Consultation with a hospitalized child is one obvious example. And, even in the hospital setting, the interviewer cannot always talk in privacy with the child in one of those small, nicely decorated rooms provided for that purpose on the wards of most hospitals. Instead, he may often find himself sitting at the bedside of an immobilized child in a room shared with three other all-eyes, all-ears children. In such a setting the interviewer cannot, obviously, give first priority to privacy. The child's scared feelings, his nightmares, his not eating, his angry thrusting aside of hypos and pills and the people who bring these things are too manifest, too immediate. The consultant has been summoned by a troubled pediatric staff, and he must do his best to talk and relate with this particular youngster in that setting. Even so, in such instances, the ward setting itself often can be utilized by the interviewer to help the bedfast child with his troubled feelings.

I recall being asked one afternoon to consult on Henry, a nine-year-old boy from a large, very poor family from the mountains of eastern Kentucky. His father had a small hillside subsistence farm and did some odd jobs. It seemed that Henry had knocked his mother's coffeepot off the stove one Saturday morning, spilling scalding coffee over much of his chest and abdomen. At the time I was asked to see him he had been on the pediatric ward of the University of Kentucky Medical Center for about five days, being treated for extensive second-degree burns. His parents and some of his other relatives had come down to Lexington to be with him. In spite of their presence, however, Henry had taken to "sulling up," as mountain people often say; he was cranky, irritable, and withdrawn to the point that he wouldn't eat, barely spoke with his kinfolk, spoke not at all with hospital personnel, and battled staff over his medications.

As I came into the room, I saw that Henry had the bed next to the window. I greeted the three other boys as I walked by them. One was about twelve; the other two appeared to be Henry's age. Henry was covered up with a burn tent from the neck down. He lay on his back, his face framed by a mass of tousled, carrot-red hair. His mouth was set in a grim line. Large freckles, made more prominent by his paleness, stood out over his face like raisins in a cake. All in all, Henry looked both angry and scared. I took a chair at the head of his bed, between him and the adjacent twelve-year-old. I told Henry I was a worry-doctor, interested in the worries and difficulties all boys have growing up, and that his regular doctor thought he had been having some worries since he had been here in the hospital and therefore wanted me to come by to talk with him. I next told Henry that I had never met him before and therefore must be a stranger to him, and as I said this he rolled over, turning his face to the wall by the window. He said nothing.

I waited quietly for a few minutes. Meanwhile, I could feel the eyes of the other three boys on the back of my neck. Then I began talking at some length about the fact that I had spoken with Henry's folks out in the lobby. They were Collettes, I told Henry I had learned, from around Lockard's Creek in Estill County. I told him of my familiarity with the area, including enough detail of people and places to make my remarks believable. At this point the twelve-year-old boy piped up eagerly, saying he knew Tracy Napier, a second cousin of his on his daddy's side, who farmed the bottomland at the mouth of Buzzard's Branch, apparently two hollows over from where the Collettes lived. "Buddy," the twelve-year-old continued, "hit sure is somethin' to wind up here in the hospital right next to a neighbor! But I sure didn't know it! That boy there hain't said six things since he's been here. Hit's a shame, too. His name's Henry, though. I'm right about that 'cause I heared his daddy call him that t'other day. His mamaw's been here, too. But she can't get nuthin' out of him, either. He's just too plumb skeered, buddy, way I figger hit. And his folks are sure skeered, too. They come in here and cry and pet on him somethin' awful!''

Led on by the twelve-year-old boy, who turned out to be Sammy Napier, I shifted from talking to turned-over Henry, and guessing out loud how he might naturally be feeling as a burned boy in a strange hospital among strangers, to talking with Sammy himself for the next twenty minutes. Sammy proved to be a very feeling-oriented boy, showing a capacity shared by many Appalachian children. What helped me most that afternoon was his marvelous ability, without much prompting from me, to put his feelings into words: "Now, take me, Doc. I been here 'bout a week, I reckon. Come here before Henry. Didn't get burned like him, though. Me and my buddies, we went over by the creek to cook some 'taters. Wood was wet, so buddy, I got some gas from my daddy's car and *whoosh*! Hit was a sight to see! Come up all over my hand, that fire did! Hit skeered me somethin' awful, I can tell you! But hit's a sight better now. Henry, there, I can't rightly tell what come over him, though. That there tent hides him so nobody can tell what really happened. Must be pretty awful, way he's kivered up!''

At this point, Henry rolled over to us abruptly. With tears welling up in his eyes, he angrily spat out: "Well, you-all ain't so much! A little bitty thing you got! 'Tain't nuthin'!'' Then Henry broke down and cried, whereupon I indicated with a jerk of my head that Sammy was to get out of bed and come over to join me at Henry's bedside. Sammy's own story had uncorked Henry's feelings. I hoped, too, that Sammy might now help Henry realize the healing process that burns go through. It did turn out that way; Sammy did a marvelous job. "Henry, I sure 'nuff did cry when I got fire on my hand—hit skeered me so. Buddy, let me see what hit done to you.'' Henry stopped openly crying, snuffled a bit, and nodded glumly. Quite gently, Sammy rolled back the covers from Henry's tent. He gasped: "Whee-you! Buddy, what in tarnation you done to get all that?'' Henry's head was up at this point, and he propped himself up further on his elbows. Then he poured out to Sammy the whole story of his spilling coffee on himself and how frightened he was, and said that for days he had imagined he was going to die, especially since his kinfolk wrung their hands and cried over him when they were in the room. In effect, Henry and Sammy were "consensually validating" each other's misfortunes and feelings.

After Henry finished, I joined Sammy, who was still looking down at the large burned patch over most of the front of Henry's chest. I pointed out to Sammy the new pink skin forming around the edges of the burn, and told the boy how this entire area would gradually heal in a similar manner. Henry was obviously interested, too. He craned his neck to see what we were talking about. Together, Sammy and I got Henry into a position to see this for himself. Henry seemed relieved. I talked further with both boys about the time it takes for full recovery from a burn and how medications help this, and said I would talk some with Henry's folks so that they could figure this whole thing out right for themselves, too. The interview ended on a recovery note: all three of us were swapping yarns about boyish wanderings in our respective woods. From then on, Henry presented no real problems on the ward.

The conclusion I drew from this experience is that there are many natural elements of a hospital setting—including, first and foremost, the other children on the ward—that can be mobilized to assist the troubled child to recognize and to ventilate his fears, and to enable him to assess what healing properties he has in himself. These elements need not present obstacles to his work, as one might expect, but can enable the consultant to work more effectively with children in the hospital setting.

THE OFFICE SETTING

The stories of Tim and Henry illustrate that occasionally, for a number of reasons, the person evaluating the troubled child must leave his office to meet the child where he is. Tim's doubts and fears—so palpable in that first, tormented interview in my office—pointed up the necessity of my home visit with him. Henry, of course, was flat on his back in a hospital.

In both cases, I reaped definite advantages from these circumstances, as would often be the case.

Generally, however, factors of time and distance work against our leaving our offices to make such visits. Furthermore, most of the time it isn't necessary: the stories, feelings, and observations shared with us by the child's parents, teachers, and so on, plus our own impressions of his functioning, give us sufficient data to enable us to do a reasonable job of evaluating the child in an office setting. But it is true that an office interview, because it takes the child out of his natural habitat, is in that way an artificial event. This artificiality may at first lead the child to relate quite differently with us from the ways he relates with other people. And what he tells us explicitly about himself may likewise be distorted, an out-of-focus picture of his functioning outside the office. It is not that we cannot work with such distortions or unclear pictures. In fact, correcting distortions and getting a child's functioning into clearer focus is a major task of ongoing treatment interviews. But it is imperative that when meeting with children we keep in mind this artificiality imposed by the interview itself, so that we can properly assess the data and impressions we obtain.

This point was vividly reconfirmed for me in a story about one of her clients told recently by Mrs. Eleanor Kelly, a psychiatric social worker at Rollman Psychiatric Institute in Cincinnati. Martha Shulte, a willowy blonde eleven-year-old, had been brought to the outpatient department at Rollman's. Mrs. Kelly met initially with the girl's parents in a joint interview to gain some understanding of the problems Martha might be having. The mother, particularly, was greatly upset over her daughter's endless dawdling over every task, from finishing the peas on her plate to going up to bed on time. Everything turned into a pitched battle that left Mrs. Shulte frustrated and furious. "Sometimes," she said, "I get the feeling she gets a kick out of getting me so upset. I have to stand over her on everything! I tell her when to do her homework, when to do the dishes. And do you think I get any cooperation from that girl? No! She sulks and pouts and throws a tantrum! Or, worse still, she acts so often like she doesn't hear me. I usually have to say something over and over again before she listens, and then only after I'm mad and yelling."

Actually, the pain Mrs. Shulte was feeling in her chronic

struggles with Martha did not prompt the family's coming to Mrs. Kelly. Instead, the child had been referred for evaluation by her very puzzled and somewhat exasperated homeroom teacher. Mrs. Kelly talked with this woman at length one evening over the telephone. Martha, it seemed, was doing as much procrastinating in the classroom as she was at home. She chronically failed to complete assignments when left on her own. Whenever her teacher spoke with her she passively blocked out directions, failing to hear them. Her oppositional behavior was never more overt than that, however. She was not considered to have major behavior problems at school. Her teacher summed up her feelings to Mrs. Kelly: "What puzzles me so, and irritates me, too, is that Martha just tunes me out."

As Mrs. Kelly talked further with the parents, she found evidence from what they said and from the ways they related with each other and with her in the interview that Mrs. Shulte was a domineering, controlling woman whose need to regulate and to watch Martha every step of the way had its own antecedents in her personal background. The family's troubles were due, in part, to Mrs. Shulte's ignorance of how her controlling ways contributed to Martha's oppositional behavior, and in part to Mr. Shulte's silent, passive, and somewhat peripheral position in the family. He took to ducking behind his newspaper, with a beer, in front of the television set while his wife and Martha controlled and counter-controlled, struggled and counter-struggled with each other.

On the basis of all these data, Mrs. Kelly anticipated meeting a sulky, pouting, perhaps even openly rebellious Martha in their first interview. Instead, when alone with Mrs. Kelly, Martha presented an altogether different picture of herself. She related as a sweet, cooperative, compliant child who seemed quite at ease as she talked on at length about her interests and hobbies. Even in fielding questions Mrs. Kelly put to her about her family and her relationships with them, Martha remained relatively unruffled. She openly denied the existence of problem areas or difficulties at home, painting instead a rosy picture of the way everyone got along. What puzzled Mrs. Kelly particularly was the lack of any open feeling of anxiety, sadness, disappointment, or anger in Martha as she spoke about her family. Nor did Martha's behavior in the interview suggest that she was experiencing any of these feelings within herself. Mrs. Kelly was stumped at the end of that first interview. Instead of the oppositional little girl she had expected to meet, she found a verbally open, well-related, altogether pleasant child.

But what was really striking about this story was Mrs. Kelly's unique way of handling, or structuring, her second evaluation interview with Martha, held a week after their first meeting. At the beginning of that second interview, the two exchanged a number of pleasantries. In fact, Mrs. Kelly felt that Martha was genuinely glad to see her again. A positive relationship between them had apparently begun to develop. Then Mrs. Kelly asked Martha to play a special kind of game with her. Martha was pleased and clapped her hands. Games were fun, she said. Mrs. Kelly explained: "Martha, this game is to be something like school. I'd like you to sit across the room from me, in that chair, with your back to me during the game. Take this tablet and pen and number every second line of your paper. Number from one to ten." Martha looked somewhat per-plexed, but quietly did as she had been instructed. Continuing, Mrs. Kelly said: "Go over now and sit with your back to me, Martha. The game is that I'll tell you to write down something by each number. I'll go slowly so you will have time to write down what I tell you to do. But I will speak only once for each number. So you must listen very, very carefully. And I will jump around. I won't take the numbers in order. Do you understand these directions for the game?" Martha nodded silently from her chair. "Now, Martha, write your father's first name on line seven." A pause, then: "Write down the numbers from eight to sixteen on line four—. Write your teacher's full name on line ten—. Write your favorite food on line five—. Write your name on line one—. Write the name of your favorite sport on line six."

And so it went, for approximately ten minutes. At the end of the game, Mrs. Kelly said: "Okay, Martha, you may turn around now. Let me see how you did." Pale, anxious, with tears in her eyes, Martha turned and offered the tablet to Mrs. Kelly. Half of the written items were missing, or were incor-rect in some manner. Martha had put in her brother's name for her father's, for example, or she had mixed up the lines. Tearfully, and then with an anxious push of speech, the child poured out: "I like you, Mrs. Kelly, I really do. I did so want to get it all right for you. But I couldn't seem to hear. I mean, I could hear, but I couldn't follow you. I got all nervous and scared. Then I got sort of frozen up inside, like I do at school when my teacher tells me to do something. I miss the directions then, and I get it all wrong if I go on. So I freeze up and don't finish anything. It's awful! The kids think I'm stupid, and now I think maybe I really am. My folks sure think so, anyway." By now, anger was beginning to give an edge to Martha's voice. "Mother especially says so, Mrs. Kelly. She's always on me for something, pushing me all the time!" Martha dissolved into sobs. As Mrs. Kelly patted her gently and got out her Kleenex for Martha, she said: "I'm really very sorry you've had to feel this way for so long, and in here again today. But I am so very glad you were willing to play a game with me that shows me very clearly just what happens at school, and how you really feel inside. I had to know that to help you."

The initial conclusion Mrs. Kelly drew from her first interview experience with Martha was that the girl genuinely liked her from the outset. Perhaps Martha's being so pleasant, so cooperative, and so well-mannered that first hour was due, at least in part, to a wish not to jeopardize this newfound, untested relationship with a woman. Certainly Mrs. Kelly must immediately have come across to Martha as a quiet, kindly person who was sincerely trying to understand how she was feeling. But the additional determinant was that the two essential elements—person and place—of Mrs. Kelly's meeting with Martha in her office combined to produce a level of artificiality that served, that first time, to obscure rather than to reveal Martha's true feelings. The office setting was not the scene where an unending number of bedtime battles were fought between Martha and her mother, nor was it the classroom in which the child tuned out her teacher. And not only was the office a sort of quiet haven away from these struggles; it also came equipped with a lady whose life-style was markedly different from her mother's.

It was no wonder, then, that Mrs. Kelly felt a special approach was necessary; she realized that one way she could see how Martha really felt and coped with problems was to structure the second evaluation hour the way she did. Her strategy demonstrated clearly how it is sometimes possible to overcome the factor of artificiality imposed by one's meeting with a child in an office setting by, in a sense, recreating a fragment of the real world of the child within the interview itself. There are many other ways of attempting to assist the child to reveal himself, of course. Another evaluator, for example, when faced with a relatively nonproductive interview as Mrs. Kelly was with Martha, might well have elected to put all three family members together in a joint interview. Onstage together, Martha and her parents would probably soon have revealed how they interacted much of the time at home! Some of these other ways are discussed in later chapters of this book which consider further practical ways of helping children alone (or a family as a whole) to tell us and show us their hopes and fears and, in so doing, to see themselves as they really are. This act of revelation, of "seeing the light," is the very heart of an evaluation of a child and his family.

TWO KEY POINTS

Whether the child is interviewed in the evaluator's office, at home, or in a special setting such as a hospital, there are two points of basic importance.

(1) The first, and most obvious, factor is the interpersonal one. The interviewer and child, together, gradually become engaged in meeting and talking with one another. Nothing is more central or more critical in the interviews than the participants themselves. As they meet and begin to relate, the interviewer is interested (a) in carefully *listening* to what the child may say about his thoughts, feelings, and behavior and (b) in carefully *observing* for feelings. The two gradually get so caught up in this process that, in time, other elements of the interview setting become extraneous. Obviously this kind of relationship can be achieved virtually anywhere, so that any spot will do, at times, for a diagnostic interview.

(2) The second crucial factor is that nowhere does a child more naturally and, therefore, more clearly reveal himself than in his accustomed surroundings—at home with his family, with his friends, and at school. Thus, were we always able to do it, we would obtain the clearest picture of a child's

functioning if we observed him in these natural settings. Occasionally, we obtain a clearer picture of a particular child when, as with Tim and Henry, circumstances literally force us out of our offices. On other occasions, we may elect to visit a child in his home or to observe at school to clarify our views of him. But again, as Mrs. Kelly demonstrated with Martha, we can generally be successful in the offices to which practical circumstances tend to confine us—if we are willing to use the ingenuity our clients have the right to expect from us.

Chapter 4.

Meeting the Family: The First Interview

Tom and Alice Russell were on time for their joint appointment with me on October 12. We met in my office two days after Mrs. Russell had called about their seven-year-old son Charlie. Both of them made rather striking first impressions. A tall, lanky, athletic man, Tom was flushed with what seemed to be embarrassment as I greeted them in the waiting room. As he helped his wife remove her coat, he made a few falsely hearty, half-joking comments about the unseasonably wet weather we were having that fall. In an effort to put Tom more at ease, I spoke briefly about the effect all the recent rain had had on my fall vegetable garden. "So you're a home gardener, too," Tom responded, some real interest mixed with relief in his voice.

As we moved together into my office, Tom and I exchanged further comments about gardening. The three of us settled into chairs. Alice, an attractive, brown-haired woman of twenty-nine, was almost dwarfed by her thirty-one-year-old husband. She watched him carefully, somewhat anxiously, as we continued to talk about our gardens. Finally, saying that she appreciated my effort to put them at ease, Alice interrupted us: "Dr. Looff, you and Tom could probably go on planting fall kale and winter radishes all morning. But Charlie's such a problem I've got to get my oar in here, too." She went on to say that coming to see me had not been easy for Tom. "If it weren't for his help Charlie would really have me backed into a corner, but he's more at home selling farm machinery or playing basketball for the men's team at our church than talking to you. I'm nervous, too, but I guess it's the same here as it usually is at home, or when we go out for an evening. Tom sort of depends on me to do much of the talking." In response to what his wife had said, Tom shifted rather nervously in his chair. But then he threw her a fond glance. With further relief in his voice he said, "Alice is right. I'm just not used to talking much about this sort of thing. "But give me a John Deere tractor to sell and I'm at home. Anyway, I know planting gardens in here won't set Charlie straight. Maybe Alice could go on telling you about him, and I'll chime in with my two bits' worth along the way."

The Spontaneous Interview. Rather quickly the Russells revealed themselves to be a stable, insightful, feeling-oriented couple who supported one another in those difficult first few minutes. This way of relating together proved to be an invaluable aid throughout this interview and our subsequent sessions. It made history taking easy. Furthermore, they were able to experience feelings connected with the events they began to describe. And both Alice and Tom really needed very little support and questioning from me to put those feelings into words. Alice led the way in describing the problems they were having with seven-year-old Charlie.

The boy, she said, was a real Jekyll-and-Hyde, "sweet and likable" one hour and a devil the next. Mrs. Snyder, the second-grade teacher, had called the parents in because Charlie was not completing any of his papers. She passed out seatwork, but instead of staying put and getting to work, Charlie went into action. "Mrs. Snyder says he wiggles around for a few minutes, and then he sings or hums, and that distracts the other children around him. Once he notices he's got their attention, oh boy! He really rolls into an act!

"Apparently he jumped up on his desk the other day and shouted that he was going to take over the spelling lesson. Before Mrs. Snyder could stop him he was shouting out words for the kids to spell—words like Pleistocene, Cenozoic, and Brontosaurus. Charlie's got this thing on right now about ancient history and the dinosaur age. He saw a *National Geographic* special on television about some of that, and he reads the *Geographic* magazines we get. But that's no excuse not to sit still and finish his spelling."

There were problems at home, too. "Why, just the other

day," Mrs. Russell said, "he stabbed his sister with the scissors
—grazed her here in her side—just because she wouldn't sit still
and play school with him! Seems like he has a one-track mind
and wants his own way in nearly everything! Elizabeth's only
four, Dr. Looff. Charlie shouldn't expect her to sit there for
an hour, playing school and spelling big words like he can.
Tom and I know he's bright. You have to be pretty sharp to
read so well and spell so well. But we know other kids who
are bright, too, and they're much less active than Charlie, and
not as distractible as he is, either. Then there are those black
furies, the moods he gets into if you thwart him in anything!"

Alice paused for breath. At this point, Tom supported his
wife's emerging story by underscoring Charlie's "being real
sharp—especially in reading, spelling, and math. Actually, I
wonder if he just isn't bored with his regular school work. He
never has trouble with his work when he wants to do it. It
comes easy for him. But, like Alice says, he gets moody and
won't finish it. Then sometimes I'm not certain but what he's
just plain lazy, and Mrs. Snyder needs to crack down harder
on him. I think she misses the cue when he is about to go into
one of these take-over spells."

Alice offered rebuttal to the cracking-down idea: "We've
tried that at home and it only makes him madder. And as for
missing cues—maybe it's just me, but there's no way I can
predict when he suddenly goes into a tirade. Why, Charlie can
be playing quietly with his dog, which he dearly loves. Then,
all of a sudden, without any warning I can see, he'll bop him
one and scream at the poor thing! You know, Dr. Looff, I've
been trying to cope with problems like this in Charlie for
years—ever since he was born. Sounds funny, I know, but he's
been a management problem for me for seven years. And so
unpredictable! Really, I wonder whether he doesn't have
minimal brain damage or something. You remember the
article about brain-damaged children that came out in *Time*
magazine several months ago? When I read that, I wondered
about Charlie. He's hyperactive, distractible, impulsive, and I
guess these fury-things might be the 'emotional lability' the
article talked about. But one thing that doesn't fit. He's a very
well-coordinated boy for his age. He draws well and handles
crayons and pencils very skillfully. Tom says Charlie's got
good hand-eye coordination—enough, anyway, to catch and

throw a football real well. So maybe his problem really isn't brain damage, but an emotional one, like Mrs. Snyder suggested. We've noticed that Charlie has one of his spells when he can't have his own way.''

Together, Alice and Tom revealed how frustrated, hurt, disappointed, and occasionally overreactively angry both became at times in their attempts to manage Charlie. The boy's teachers in both kindergarten and first grade had experienced similar problems with him, but tended, they felt, to allow Charlie to drift, to have his own way. A confrontation of wills, they indicated, meant emotional fireworks! They felt that problems were coming up more often because Mrs. Snyder was a strict disciplinarian who wanted quiet among the children and no interference with her lesson plans.

Charlie's distractibility, they suggested, was in itself a variable behavior. Alice pointed out that Charlie could sit for hours in front of the television set, apparently engrossed in one of his natural science programs—"wild horses thundering by couldn't distract him at those times." Or he might sit reading a nature magazine, or spend more than an hour quietly drawing (one of his favorite pastimes). On the other hand, Tom mentioned that the boy loved playing ball with him, but that his attention span outdoors often lasted no more than five or six minutes. "We start playing okay, but a robin will fly by and he'll stop throwing the ball to notice it—with a lot of comments—or he'll see a cloud that reminds him of some long-winded story that doesn't go anywhere. You have to know how I am, Dr. Looff. I'm a now-let's-play-ball fellow all the way! So it's frustrating for me when Charlie is distracted from our game. I usually end up hollering at him, and he ends up crying to Alice. I'll admit it, she and I have had a few words over this.''

Alice confirmed that she and Tom often disagreed openly on ways to handle Charlie. She felt Tom had a tendency to leave discipline almost entirely to her, which she naturally resented. Tom tried to rationalize this tendency of his by saying that his wife was around the boy more. They did agree, after some talk, that Tom had an explosive temper, and because of this, he felt more comfortable leaving any disciplinary confrontations to Alice.

For her part, Alice—particularly over the past three years—

had grown increasingly doubtful over her ability to handle
their son at all. Nothing seemed to work, even though she was
a trained schoolteacher and should therefore, she thought, be
able to understand and handle her son. She had tried reasoning with Charlie, bribing him, screaming, and spanking. But,
she said, "the one thing I have noticed lately is that when
I send him to his room he usually settles right down and begins to read or play with his erector set or something. Even
that makes me mad, though! Here he is, enjoying being pun-
ished! I'm left shaken and angry, and he acts like it all never
happened. Some days I feel so defeated I just cry in our bed-
room for what seems like hours! And Tom and I can't even
go out anymore—Charlie's behavior has driven all our baby-
sitters away. My mother lives with us, and she's the only person who's still willing to spend some time with him. But even
she won't take him by herself. So Tom and I can't go out for
dinner and a movie, or go bowling, or visit other couples. I
feel like a prisoner in my own home." Here Alice began to
cry openly. Tom moved quickly to comfort her, and presently,
her composure restored, Alice moved on to some further
points about Charlie's behavior.

The two agreed their son, between his "furies," was a
warm, personable, altogether charming boy "with a real gift
of gab." He seemed, in their opinion, "to know no strangers.
With them, and with us too at times, he can be real likable,
friendly, and outgoing." They offered as an example how
much Charlie and his maternal grandmother enjoyed playing
chess together in her basement apartment in their home.
"Why, the two of them can sit for hours, swapping yarns."
From their story, I got the distinct impression that Charlie
was an essentially well-related youngster. Alice and Tom confirmed that Charlie related well to children his own age in the
neighborhood and, apparently, to most of those in his classroom. His warmth and outgoingness attracted other children
to him almost immediately. But sooner or later, Charlie's need
to take over a group, to be bossy and to tell everyone what to
do, got him into difficulty with the other children. As Tom
put it: "Charlie's a bosom pal for five or six minutes. Then
watch out! If the kids don't do like he says, he hits them or
has a tantrum. Either way, they go away. Then he comes in
and complains to Alice they don't like him anymore. Right

now, the kids in the neighborhood all avoid him. They steer well away. Or, they bait him to get his angry reaction." Alice and Tom indicated as well that Charlie was quite an independent fellow, with good habit patterns. He slept soundly without wetting the bed, and he managed his own dressing, eating, and toileting very well. His pediatrician had always viewed Charlie as "a healthy specimen." The boy presented no peculiar mannerisms, tics, or gestures. His verbal skills were well above those of most children his age in vocabulary level, in his general fund of information, and in the rich, abstract way he utilized language as a tool. Furthermore, they felt that he spoke clearly, articulating well without stuttering or stammering. Charlie's interests were many and varied. His interest in nature seemed deep and abiding; it was expressed through hiking, camping, watching television shows on nature themes, reading, collecting fossils, and, above all, talking—seemingly endlessly at times—about such interests. Alice was quick to point out, however, that Charlie, even in his beloved nature hobbies, was inconsistent. "He skips from one thing to another so often. Makes you dizzy sometimes! Here he's describing his rock collection to me one minute, then he goes charging off to look out the window at a tree in bloom! I'm left feeling I'm chained to the tail of Halley's comet! Dr. Looff, you can see we really do need advice about understanding Charlie. Can you help us to help him?"

At this point, the time was nearly over for that first joint interview with Charlie's parents. The Russells had in fact accomplished a great deal in outlining their son's problems to me, and in so doing they had clarified some of their views of his behavior for themselves as well. Charlie, according to the story they presented, was a bright, well-related boy. But he was also distractible, impulsive, hyperactive at times, aggressive, and often emotionally labile. Although Alice felt confused, frustrated, and often inadequate in her handling of their son over the years, she had nonetheless revealed herself to be a quite mature woman who sincerely wanted to understand and more appropriately guide Charlie. From her interview attitudes and behavior I derived no impression that Alice was an ambivalent woman, covertly or openly hostile in her relationships with either her husband or their son. With Tom she related very well indeed. Theirs seemed to be a stable marriage. And she revealed in her story that she loved Charlie but was troubled about his behavior. She did not understand the boy, and, accordingly, she could not manage him in any consistent, successful way. Furthermore, she revealed natural resentment that Tom should leave so much of Charlie's management to her. Tom, on his part, did not become defensive over his wife's revealing these feelings toward him. Instead, he supported Alice, stating that her story was accurate, and he added to it his knowledge that he tended to hand off to others problems with which he could not cope immediately because of his temper.

By their story and the sharing of their feelings, the Russells underscored again for me how significant are the complaints parents give initially and spontaneously to the interviewer. As with many parents one meets for the first time, neither of them required much verbal support from me as interviewer or from each other to continue sharing both historical and feeling data surrounding, or providing the context for, their son's problems.

Resistive Parents—the "Dental Interview." Some couples are not able to be so spontaneous in the initial, joint session, and theirs becomes what I call a "dental interview." In such cases one has to drill deeply for whatever data concerning background and feelings can be extracted. Even so, the interviewer gains much from even the most guarded, defensive, resistive parents. What is it, he asks himself, that has made them act this way? Is it individual life-styles—mistrust, suspicion, inhibitory reserve, for example—that are operating in one or both parents to retard the flow of the interview? Or might it be problems in the parents' marriage, surfacing here as a who-is-the-more-adequate-parent issue or as mutual competitiveness expressed in a minor battle for control of the interview? These are just two examples of the role behavior you may see in a couple faced with the task of cooperating to tell the interviewer about their child.

Parents can have other feelings that often put them on the defensive, at least initially, with the interviewer. A common one is guilt, often mixed with feelings of inadequacy; they have not lived up to their expectations of themselves as parents. Such feelings are betrayed frequently by their statements blaming themselves or each other for the child's problems. One way to help these parents accurately label their guilt is for the interviewer to universalize-generalize with a statement that all parents feel quite beaten down by their children's difficulties at times, to the point where they often feel powerless to handle or even understand them. The interviewer can then gently but firmly indicate that the "blaming" statements he has been hearing suggest to him that they, like many other parents, feel "blameworthy" and, no doubt, guilty and inadequate with respect to meeting their child's needs. Such an approach often helps parents feel that they are not alone with such troublesome feelings but that others have had the same difficulties. Relieved a bit, both parents may then be able to examine and accurately label inner feelings when the interviewer wonders aloud whether their "blaming" statements bespeak personal guilty feelings. Once labeled accurately, parental guilt can often be alleviated sufficiently to permit the interview to move on.

It is frequently helpful if, at this point, the interviewer indicates that he considers this talking with the child's parents to be a process in which three responsible adults are "working on a riddle together—the riddle of trying to understand, together, why the child behaves as he does." The interviewer is saying that he views the parents as perfectly adequate historians, now capable of sharing with him information on the history of their child's behavior and their feelings about it. By pointing up this concept of an interview alliance between himself and the parents, the evaluator relieves guilt further and supports them by uncovering an area in which they can express their adequacy: "So you see, Mr. and Mrs. Smith, I'm pretty much in the dark here. Your comments about your son Henry, and how he makes you feel, are the only things that can shed some light on this riddle of Henry's behavior. So please help me. Share with me what you know so well about him."

Resistive anger is another emotion which is often difficult for parents to discuss and show openly in an interview. Parents who have been forced to seek help for their child often feel angry. This may impede the progress of the diagnostic study unless the anger is accurately labeled and dealt with. The diagnostic process actually begins with the parents' decision, voluntary or forced, to seek help for the child. A beginning understanding of parental attitudes can be achieved by learning whether parents are motivated primarily by their own concern about the child or by pressures from others in the community. This includes consideration of the parents' awareness of their own involvement in the problem—whether they feel excessive guilt or self-blame or project the total responsibility onto the child, some illogical physical cause, the school, the social agency, or physicians or others who are referring sources.

The Russells came largely voluntarily, seeking help to understand Charlie. To be sure, they came at the point where behaviors similar to those they had wrestled with at home for years had nearly brought their child's expulsion from school. But they did not feel forced into coming. Instead, they agreed with the teacher that Charlie's school behavior clearly pointed up the need for evaluation. They were clearly dismayed, and often angry, over Charlie's behavior. But they were not angry with the school. This important difference in feeling enabled them to approach their initial, joint interview without feeling that they had been forced into something they did not want or feel the need for. If, however, parents are resistive in the first interview as a consequence of feeling forced into the child's evaluation, the interviewer must recognize such feelings and help the parents recognize them as well. Otherwise, there can be no real working alliance between the interviewer and the parents in the diagnostic study. This alliance is essential for an in-depth history of the child's total functioning, a revealing of all the forces that may be shaping his behavior, and the beginning of a working-together-on-the-same-riddle approach to better parental management of the child.

Within that first interview, the evaluator gains further insights concerning the parents' feelings about the child and about their own capacity to participate in the study as he begins to understand their conscious and unconscious desires and expectations for help in the diagnostic process. Apparent readiness on the parents' part may sometimes hide great resistance, which may later be reflected in the child's degree of accessibility when his turn comes to meet with the evaluator. But whether the parents reveal feelings of anxiety, self-criticism and guilt, or complete irresponsibility or hostility either to the child, the referring source, the clinic, or the evaluator, our goal is to provide understanding support to enable them to express the negative reactions which might otherwise block their participation.

By devoting time to this area of the parents' feelings at the beginning of the initial exploration of their child's problems, the evaluator can usually enable the parents to take the steps that will involve them and their child in the diagnostic process. Some of these feelings—like guilt, inadequacy, and anger —have been reviewed here. But all expressions of feeling and all observed attitudes in parents are in fact grist to the diagnostic mill; this is true as well for the parents' reaction to further office or clinic procedures undertaken in the study of their child. Variations on the feeling theme are all facets of the parents' anxieties, of their sense of failure, of their disappointments, of their hidden or manifest hostility, of their fear of being revealed through the child—as well as of their concern lest the child find in his relationship with the interviewer the satisfactions which they themselves presumably were unable to provide. By helping the parents deal with their own anxieties and misconceptions, where these exist, the interviewer lays the groundwork for the kind of relationship— a working alliance—on which comprehensive diagnosis depends.

Planning with the Parents. At the end of my initial interview with the Russells, it was apparent that we had achieved a working alliance from which we could shape Charlie's diagnostic study. Alice and Tom agreed that we needed to take enough interview time to examine carefully all the forces that might be shaping the boy's behavior. They accepted the comprehensive six-interview format, the one I had suggested to Mrs. Russell at the time of her telephone inquiry. Accordingly, at the end of that interview hour we set appointment times for Charlie's two interviews with me, times for both Alice's and Tom's individual interviews, and a time for our final, joint follow-up conference to conclude the diagnostic study.

Tom then expressed concern about the fees involved. He had, he indicated, no comprehensive medical insurance that would cover Charlie's psychiatric outpatient evaluation. As we talked about this, he said emphatically that he wanted to pay the full fee for private services, but that he would prefer to pay his bill over a year's time, in order to better budget his monthly salesman's salary. Together, we accepted this full-fee, pay-over-a-year plan. As a general rule, discussions about fees are engaged in at the end of the initial interview with the parents. They are, of course, entitled to know the charges for the diagnostic interviews then being planned. And if a good working alliance has been achieved during that initial interview, talk about fees can proceed in a climate of positive rapport. This certainly seemed to be true with the Russells.

At the very end of that first interview, I gave the Russells a copy of the *Developmental Questionnaire* (see Appendix) adapted for our use at the Child Psychiatry Clinic, University of Kentucky Medical Center, from one used for years at the Menninger Foundation.[1] They were asked to fill this out together, in order to share with me important data about Charlie's formative years. The questionnaire was explained as a homework item, a data-obtaining instrument that would save valuable interview time for the exchange of further ideas and feelings they both would have about Charlie's functioning. I asked Mrs. Russell to bring the completed questionnaire when she came for her individual interview, in order that I could review it quickly with her then and with her husband subsequently. Then they gave me permission to talk directly with Mrs. Snyder about Charlie's problems in school.

All of these final points (including the important one discussed in the next two paragraphs) having been raised and agreed upon, we closed our first interview. As Tom left the waiting room, he grinned back at me, saying, "You know, you're doing the same thing with us I do as coach with our church basketball team—diagramming all the plays on the blackboard! And I like it!"

Telling the Child. An important aspect of the six-interview plan is that the parents are launched into it before the child has his first session with the evaluator. This means that they have the opportunity to discuss with the evaluator how they should tell the child about this new experience, and they

---

1. The basic outline for our own developmental questionnaire was adapted from the one in use by the Child Psychiatry Division, The Menninger Foundation, Topeka, Kans. I am indebted to those clinicians in that group who, through the years, developed their particular form. In our own clinic, Dr. Billy Ables and Natasha Pfeiffer, M. S. W., did the major work of revision and extension of this model to produce the final form of the questionnaire we have used subsequently.

have a chance to reveal any fears they may have concerning the child's reaction to it. These are, of course, opportunities for the evaluator as much as for the parents, and a wise clinician will make full and responsible use of them.

Alice herself asked me for help in preparing Charlie for his coming to see me. Her own idea was to tell him they had already been to talk with a doctor because they were worried and upset over some of the things Charlie did, and, because they loved him, they wanted the doctor to help them understand why these things happened; they wanted the doctor's help so they could all get along better. I told Mrs. Russell this seemed a good, sensitive way to convey the meaning of the evaluation to the boy. I asked her to add to her explanation the statement that "Dr. Looff is a worry-doctor, a doctor who is interested in the worries and problems all boys and girls have growing up. And he doesn't give shots!" I explained to Mrs. Russell that I have found the phrase "worry-doctor" useful to convey to a younger child my role and functioning. The phrase "all children have growing up" conveys a universalization-generalization theme designed to offset the child's natural feeling of vulnerability at being singled out, as he might view it, from other children. Finally, the phrase "and he doesn't give shots" is to make it quite clear that coming to my office is quite different from visiting the family physician, something the young child often views, apprehensively, as an all-hypodermic experience.

Alice understood the need for these statements. "But Charlie is bright, Dr. Looff. If you don't give shots, he'll want to know just what you will do together." She was asked to explain further that as a worry-doctor, I was interested in talking over his feelings with Charlie, and that I had a special playroom in which we could talk and play together in order to get his feelings carefully understood.

THE SHORT-TERM DIAGNOSTIC-TREATMENT STUDY

The point was made earlier that the inquiry itself shapes the plan for the subsequent diagnostic study. Three types of diagnostic plans, all of which take their shape from parental inquiries, were outlined in Chapter 2. The first, that applicable to the Russell family, meets the need for a thorough diagnostic study of a child with chronic learning and behavior problems. The second, that applicable to the Shugars family, is an example of a study plan for a family having concerns about relatively selective, focused behaviors in an otherwise well-functioning child that seem amenable to short-term diagnostic-treatment interviews.

The reader will recall Mrs. Shugars's telephone inquiry about her son Chester, the four-year-old "apron-string" child whose home background appeared to fit a fairly typical picture. In cases like Chester's, where a youngster can function generally quite well except in the area of separating from his parents to master new situations independently, I have found that short-term treatment interviews focused on the family's parent-child relationships often help these parents redirect their training efforts. This is agreed on with the parents at the outset.

Evelyn Shugars's telephone call to me that particular morning near the end of May was prompted by Chester's refusal to have a Head Start physical examination by Dr. William Becknell, their family physician. This man had known Evelyn and Frank Shugars for years. Furthermore, he was well aware they were "apron-stringing" Chester. Chester's refusal to be examined led him to direct Evelyn Shugars to call me. The referral was an appropriate one, and Dr. Becknell had prepared them well for it. They anticipated receiving help from me, but held no expectations that I would magically "fix Chester." In fact, Evelyn Shugars said at the time of her inquiry: "I know we're doing something wrong. Maybe you can help set us straight." When she called me, I told Mrs. Shugars that it would help my understanding of Chester and their family if I had her permission to call Dr. Becknell directly before they came to see me. I wanted, I told her, to have a picture of them as Dr. Becknell had known them for years. She could see the value of such a call, and gave me her permission to talk with their doctor. Mrs. Shugars and I then set the date and time for my first, joint interview with them—approximately ten days from the time of her inquiry. A day or two after Mrs. Shugars called, I talked with Dr. Becknell for twenty minutes over the telephone. From what he said, the following picture took shape in my mind.

It was nine o'clock on a fine May morning in Manchester, county seat of Clay County, in eastern Kentucky. The scene was Dr. Becknell's crowded waiting room. The doctor and his brother James had been doing medical histories and physical examinations on a number of four- and five-year-old boys and girls due to enter either the local Head Start or day-care program the following month. The chorus from their waiting room was like the sounds made by a group of preschoolers and their mothers gathered anywhere else: some children, grinning, pushed and pummeled each other until shushed into momentary inactivity by their mothers; other youngsters giggled and whispered. Utilizing the long wait as a kaffeeklatsch, the mothers talked quietly with their kinfolk, friends, and neighbors. Occasionally, the children looked up when one of their number, somewhere back in an inner office, produced a brief wail over a vaccination. On the whole, however, there was very little anxiety among the children. Friendly and outgoing, the great majority of these four- and five-year-olds functioned quite well on their own, meeting and mastering their feelings at being examined by the physicians.

Then the waiting-room picture changed quite suddenly. Plump, ample Evelyn Shugars, thirty-two, her face flushed with physical effort and the unexpressed tension and frustrated anger she felt, came in dragging her four-year-old Chester by the hand. Chester had a round, full face, no neck—his head screwed down between wide shoulder blades—his sturdy trunk and legs braced firmly against his mother's dragging. He was obviously pouting, a lip "a frog could sit on" thrust forward beneath firmly knit eyebrows. In his free hand he clutched a bottle of strawberry pop, a bag of potato chips, and an all-day sucker. The receptionist was told by tense-angry Evelyn that these were bribes she had used to get Chester that far.

That the mother as well as Chester had difficulties separating in order to master the examination situation became painfully evident within minutes of their arrival. Dr. Becknell, alerted by his nurse that there was potential trouble in the waiting room, attempted to see them ahead of the others. Although he explained the procedures in a friendly, easy-going manner, Chester bawled, "I don' wanna—I don' wanna!" and plastered himself to Evelyn's coat. With mounting tension in her voice, she struggled to pull the boy free from her. "It's so embarrassing, doctor. Every time we go anywhere it's the same thing—he just can't do anything on his own. I've got to be right there! You'd think once in a while he'd do what he's supposed to do! I've told him that you'd just hurt him a little bit!" At this statement, delivered as it was with Evelyn's wavering anxiety, Chester began a screaming, foot-stamping tantrum. The boy, bright and sensitive to feelings in others, was clearly tuned in to his mother's vacillation in the situation. Evelyn's anxieties spilled over even more. She pushed Chester toward Dr. Becknell and exploded: "By God, Chester, if you don't go with the doctor I'll have him give you two shots!" The boy stopped screaming, clutched at his mother and burst into tears. "You don' wuv me—you don' wuv me anymore!" With this guilt-instilling technique, Chester brought down what little angry resolve Evelyn may have possessed for a moment. She picked him up and tried to soothe him. "There, there, don't cry. Mommy didn't mean to upset you."

Obviously, no one was in a frame of mind to pursue the examination. With one eye on his knowledge of the Shugars family and their ways of relating with Chester, Dr. Becknell decided that the time had clearly come to help the parents, if possible, to redirect their training efforts with their son. Knowing that he did not have the interview time to do this just then, Dr. Becknell decided on the spot—utilizing the mother's conflicted feelings in his office—to refer her to me. He suggested gently but firmly that she and Frank, her husband, contact me at one of our field clinics for child psychiatry at the local health department. A dependent woman, faced also with her torment of the moment with Chester, Mrs. Shugars accepted the referral.

The Family Interview—Background. Frank and Evelyn, with Chester again in reluctant tow, came in to see me several days later. In an attempt to round out the situation for the boy I told him about my role as a "worry-doctor." The family was interviewed jointly. While Frank, Evelyn, and I talked, Chester played on the floor with a few toys in a plastic basin. From time to time he looked up, seeming to tune in quite well to our discussion.

As we talked, both Frank and Evelyn showed themselves to

be bright, concerned, overanxious parents who really wanted advice on how to help Chester. Both were stocky, moderately obese people who clearly doted on the boy, their only child, and were intensely wrapped up in his care. Gradually, the story emerged that began to explain Chester's failure to achieve the degree of autonomy appropriate to his age (reflected in the boy's poor capacity to separate from either one of his parents), his marked shyness at times (clinging to his mother's side) and overdependence on them, and his immaturely aggressive temper tantrums.

Frank and Evelyn pointed out that Chester was always particularly anxious on occasions demanding some separation from them, as in Dr. Becknell's office. At these times he became whining, demanding, and clinging, and alternatively was shy and withdrawn and displayed temper tantrums. What also emerged—and here both parents were open and honest about their feelings and behavior toward Chester—was a clear picture of how each of them had infantilized, hovered over, and overprotected the boy from birth on. This constant babying seemed to act as a powerful model for the boy's infantile behavior. But why had Frank and Evelyn directed Chester's growth in this manner? As we talked further, some determinants of their behavior came to light.

First of all, both Frank and Evelyn were raised in large, close-knit, inner-directed families typical of the Southern Appalachian region. As children of poor but stable working-class families who managed to eke out an existence on small subsistence farms, Chester's parents from their infancy were raised in a particular type of regional training climate. They, like many other children in the area, were taught in verbal and nonverbal ways to maintain the close family system itself, even at the expense of their own personal and social maturation. Evelyn recalled in our interview, for example, that her mother taught her to stay close through the psychology of fear: "Stay right here, Evie, or I'll leave you!" Thus their own growth and development as children were clearly subordinated to the prime task of maintaining the family as a close unit. This fostering of family closeness was understandable in a mountainous region where families faced on their own the harsh facts of geographic isolation in coves and hollows, poverty, underemployment, and chronic ill health in many family members—stresses that would make those of any television soap-opera family mild by comparison. In the past there were no viable social institutions outside the family that could effectively assist them with their burdens. This cultural fact forced families to turn inward upon themselves to face problems as best they could from a position of family solidarity.

But for Frank and Evelyn, as for many children growing up in the Southern Appalachian region, there were both positive and negative effects of such a close system. On the positive side, families got together for big dinners and reunions, and often came long distances back home to share themselves and their meager resources at times of need or crisis. The negative effect, which we often saw operating at the clinic in families like the Shugarses, was the threat that the independent, autonomous functioning of any one person posed to the integrity of the family as a whole. This threat was clearly seen in the great frequency with which separation anxiety was the emotional conflict faced by children and by their families. Of all their troubles, disruptions in parent-child and other family relationships—whether actual, threatened, or symbolic—caused them the most concern. Thus it was that Frank and Evelyn, like many other people in their area, brought to their marriage trained-in concerns about keeping families close and avoiding separation at all costs. But, as it turned out, such feelings were not alone responsible for their hovering overprotection of Chester; other determinants of their behavior came to light as we talked further.

At the time they were married, Evelyn was sixteen and in her junior year of high school. Frank, three years older, had finished the eighth grade and was already well established as a finishing carpenter. For a time after they married they wanted no children. Frank worked regularly, Evelyn got a job in a beauty parlor, and they, with others, enjoyed late adolescent fun and games. A year later, however, they actively wanted a child of their own. For the next ten years they worked at it with consistent effort but no success. Frank, it finally turned out on examination, had a low sperm count, and Evelyn, as she put it, "had collapsed tubes." It was after much sexual counseling, and tubal insufflation of Evelyn, that they conceived Chester. Both of them recalled in our interview how ecstatic they felt during the pregnancy.

The Shugarses obviously thought of Chester as God's very special gift to them. They told me of his infancy in great detail: every burp, gurgle, coo, bath, diaper, and feeding brought them very great pleasure as they sketched in the boy's early history. Apparently, their relationships with him were highly permissive and indulgent. For example, on nights when Chester seemed fussy about going off to sleep, one of them would lie down with him, sometimes for hours, until he fell asleep. And, when he was old enough for finger foods at the table, Evelyn was quite content to go on feeding him herself. The boy took a night-time bottle until he was three and a half. As Evelyn put it: "We didn't want to deprive him of something he seemed to enjoy and wanted so much." As it turned out, Chester was the one who finally threw the bottle away. Thus, both in what they were saying about Chester as an infant and in the pleasure-filled manner with which they presented such data, Frank and Evelyn underscored how freely they had given of themselves to Chester, who as an infant seemed to thrive in every way.

But beginning with the motor-muscular (after eighteen months) and preschool stages of development of the boy, Frank's and Evelyn's attitudes as parents began to interfere with Chester's ability to gain independence, to achieve emerging autonomy through doing certain self-help tasks for himself. When Chester attempted to toddle off, they overprotectively called him back to be near them. He was not allowed, for example, to ride his tricycle in the driveway "because the coal trucks might run him over" (the main road was a half-mile away). He was cautioned out of climbing lest he fall and hurt his head. Furthermore, when he responded to their entreaties to stay close, they both displayed the indulgent, permissive behavior they had shown toward him as an infant. Chester in turn reacted to this overprotectiveness and infantilization with similar modes of adjustment—clinging, whining, demanding, and basking in being babied. Similarly, the parents set very few disciplinary limits. When they did— and these were set inconsistently—Chester reacted with temper tantrums. They then fed these tantrums by yielding, as Evelyn had done in Dr. Becknell's office by bribing the boy and by excusing him from the examination task at hand.

What seemed to be the case was that the Shugarses, both

because of their trained-in attitudes about family closeness and because of the specific difficulty they had had in bearing a child, saw Chester's emerging autonomy as a threat to their complete domination and possession of him. They dealt with this threat by intensifying their overprotection and infantilization of him. "We wanted him so much. He was such a long time coming. And we wanted him to have an easier life than we had as kids. Maybe we have spoiled him. The neighbors think so, anyway. But it's hard to let him go. Suppose something awful happened to him, like getting hurt! And really, doctor, it's our pleasure to do for him as long as he's at home." How revealing were these words, providing as they did a full picture of their feelings about Chester and about their rearing of him.

It is possible for the primary physician to undertake a program of direct intervention with the family of an apron-string child, before the problem becomes severe enough to warrant referral to a mental health clinic. Sometimes, however, as with the Shugarses, the physician has spotted the problem but simply doesn't have the time for interviews with the family. Prompt referral to a mental health clinic then is appropriate. Our clinic experience with such families is outlined here as one model for effective local treatment. The plan is set in motion at the time of the first, joint meeting with the family. The model has been used successfully by several physicians, psychologists, social workers, public health nurses, and mental health associates in areas in rural Kentucky, and I have employed it in a child psychiatry clinic setting and in private practice.

Aims and Techniques of Short-term Treatment. The overall goal is to utilize the pain—the feelings of frustration, embarrassment, guilt, anxiety, and anger—that parents feel when their child cannot function on his own as a lever to move them to redirect their training efforts with him. Parents would like to avoid such painful feelings, if possible, so it is with these feelings that the interviewer should begin.

The feelings will emerge naturally if the interviewer insists that, in his initial interview, both the parents and the child be present. This puts them all on stage, doing what comes naturally. Within minutes of my seeing the Shugarses together, for example. Chester had literally hog-tied his mother with his demanding whining. She began to feed him bubble gum in an effort to silence him. This brought flushed anger to Mr. Shugars's face; he knew his wife was behaving inappropriately, but he felt powerless to intervene. So that in future interviews the discussion will be able to develop as fruitfully as possible, we have often followed the practice of not having the child back after this first joint interview. He is in there just once, to mobilize pain in his parents and to give the interviewer an opportunity to see in what ways the parents behave appropriately and in what ways inappropriately toward him.

As part of his initial assessment of the entire family's weaknesses and strengths, the interviewer determines two points of critical importance:

(1) The degree of emotional separation of parents and child. This is judged by their history as well as by their reaction to the current crisis (school examination for Chester). It is a sign of relative strength in both if the child is struggling against his fears of separation (Chester sometimes did want to ride his trike alone), and if the mother and father still attempt to have the child function apart from them despite his discomfort (it was a strength in Evelyn that she had dragged Chester to the examination after deciding that she wanted him in the Head Start program, even though she later gave up trying for the moment). It is a less promising sign if both have given up trying to be separated.

(2) The degree of the parents' anger toward their child. A very favorable sign is the mother's ability to express her annoyed frustration over the situation, to express anger toward her child openly and without crippling guilt ("By God, Chester!"). By contrast, the apathetically resigned mother who cannot protest the situation is difficult to mobilize toward firm limit setting.

The mother's frustrated anger is a most helpful feeling. It is the force the interviewer uses to prod her in the direction of firmness with the child. Some mothers need the interviewer's active permission (granted through his role as an authority figure for the family) to be openly angry with their children. Such mothers are either guilty about their anger or feel that being firm is a hostile act that will cause their children not to love them anymore (Evelyn so often felt this way

that Chester had seized on "you don' wuv me" as a very effective, guilt-instilling technique that tore down his mother's resolve where any limits were concerned). The interviewer here,
while at the same time universalizing-generalizing that any
mother would be angry when her child behaves in such an infantile manner, relieves guilt: "It's okay, Evelyn, to let Chester
see you're mad. You can tell him that you'll always love him,
but there are certain things he does that make you mad, behaviors that just don't go." By doing this, the interviewer re-
directs the mother's anger from previous impotent rages that
led nowhere to directed firmness in setting needed limits.

The interviewer also clarifies for the parents the relative
part cultural or specific family factors may have played in
their overprotection and infantilization of the child: "Since
you waited ten years for Chester, I can see in one way how
much you'd want to watch out for him." Another approach
the interviewer can use when the mothers and fathers vacillate
in setting limits is to remind them of the pain they've felt in
the past. To avoid future pain they often are ready, with the
interviewer's constant emotional support and encouragement,
to begin setting limits with the child.

Early in short-term treatment one cannot expect the parents
to want separated functioning of the child as a developmental
goal for its own sake. That realization will only come later
when, with the child functioning on his own at least some of
the time, they feel better, are more in control of the child, and
discover that he still loves them. The interviewer's first step
is to relieve the parents of painful feelings. Only later will they
have feelings of satisfaction gained from helping their child to
function autonomously.

Practical Steps. By using these feeling-oriented approaches
—reinforced by his seeing the parents briefly each week if
possible—the interviewer can, in a relatively short time, go
over practical steps they can take to help their child to separate. Self-help tasks are discussed, as well as the importance
of firm, kind, consistent limit setting. Occasions for the child
to function separately—riding a tricycle, staying for an afternoon with a friend's child in their home, joining a nursery or
a day-care peer group—are carefully looked for as opportunities for him to practice emerging skills and freedoms. Where

they succeed, parents are warmly praised by the interviewer. When they vacillate, he reminds them again of pain. The parents and the interviewer know when gradual progress is being made. It is a favorable sign when both parents and child use the support offered by the interviewer to separate increasingly. Furthermore, the decline in the parents' overprotectiveness and infantilization, which fosters the child's increasing independence, is accompanied by marked positive changes in feelings in family members. Together they begin to like "having more room to move around in," as the Shugarses summarized the progress they made with Chester.[2]

THE APPROACH TO A FAMILY IN CRISIS

Example of a First Interview and the Patterns It Reveals. The two types of diagnostic study described so far are both shaped by the parents' initial inquiry. This is true as well for studies involving families in some sort of emotional crisis. If the parent who calls is distressed because of a school-phobic reaction,[3] a suicidal attempt, or acutely antisocial and self-destructive behavior like fire-setting, stealing, drug abuse, sexual promiscuity, or running away from home, I treat the problem as an emergency. Accordingly, I plan that the first interview—set for that day, if possible, or certainly no later than the next— include both parents and the child in joint session. Often, particularly in crises involving an adolescent, I ask the family to bring with them an older sibling if there is one. This person often functions usefully as a "predictor," that is, a more objective ego-observer of the family's problems, of their traditional ways of coping with stress, and of their ego strengths. The family in their initial interview are put together, onstage as it were, to reveal ideas, feelings, and ways of relating together. This information is essential for crisis resolution, for planning for short-term management procedures, and for outlining further diagnostic-treatment sessions.

2. Looff, "The Apron-String Child."
3. David H. Looff, "School Phobia in the Southern Appalachian Region: Crucial Importance of Early Treatment," *Southern Medical Journal*, 62, No. 3, March 1969, pp. 329-35.

An example of an interview with a family in crisis was furnished by Pete, an adolescent, and his divorced mother. This woman, Mrs. Woodridge, called because Pete's school principal had suspended him for chronic truancy and for breaking some light fixtures in the cafeteria immediately after he had been bawled out for being absent so much. The principal had told Pete's mother the boy would not be permitted to return to school until he had had a psychiatric evaluation. I met with Pete and his mother jointly the day following her call.

In the waiting room, and throughout much of the initial part of the joint interview, fourteen-year-old Pete slouched sullenly in his chair. Both his long hair and his blue denim clothes were dirty. He glowered at his mother, without saying anything, during her long recitals of his sins. At other times he smoked cigarettes nervously, yet insolently, dangling them from the corner of his mouth. Mrs. Woodridge, thirty-two, was a tense, angry, careworn, chronically depressed woman who in dramatic, martyred words told how life had been one heavy burden for her. First, there was her chronically unemployed husband, who, when drunk, had hurled profane remarks at her and cuffed her about throughout the first sixteen years of a miserable marriage. Two years ago, she indicated, he had finally run off to Ohio with his most recent mistress. Every other weekend her husband returned to the family's small hillside farm in rural Kentucky to spree-drink with his coon-hunting cronies, to cuff her about some more, and to have his laundry done. Mrs. Woodridge clearly seemed adept at creating problems for herself. She had not been able to take one step to begin to improve the marriage, or, failing this, to terminate it. Nor could she stop darkly predicting that Pete would, in all probability, grow up—as she told me there in the interview in Pete's presence—"to be a bastard just like his old man." When she made such comments, Pete was moved to angry rebuttal. It was clear, from the way they related in the interview, that at home Pete flared up repeatedly in response to his mother's critical, disparaging, provocative comments.

As they talked, I learned that, as a child, Pete would cry when his father was gone or when his mother lashed out critically at either of them. As an early adolescent, Pete had stopped crying. Instead, he had begun to snarl back at his mother, and, by displacement, at his teachers and younger brother and two sisters. Mrs. Woodridge in turn had taken this behavior to indicate she had been right all along—Pete was no good at all. Gradually, he had lost interest in his studies and become increasingly truant from school.

As their anguished story unfolded, I could see that Pete was, underneath his sullenness and bravado, a reasonably warm, well-related youth. He also was representative of a large number of generally older adolescent boys who are referred to child psychiatry clinics with a variety of symptoms, usually chronic learning and behavior problems related to underlying difficulties in establishing a comfortable identity as a developing man. These youngsters do not develop conversion reactions, anxiety attacks, or other neurotic symptoms. Instead, they act out their feelings of inadequacy as boys, or their low self-regard, in some form of chronic misbehavior.

In general, the training influences in the lives of these acting-out adolescents are similar to those for boys with anxious-dependent personalities. As with the latter group, boys like Pete who have oppositional personality disorders generally have been raised from early childhood by women alone. Their fathers have died, deserted their families, or divorced their wives; men have been virtually absent from the developmental picture. Boys in both groups often have had several older women as training models—widowed maternal grandmothers, their own mothers, and sometimes older sisters. In addition to anxious and dependent character traits, the effeminacy of some of these boys marks the extent of their psychosexual confusion, and their difficulties in establishing appropriate sex-role behavior as adolescent boys underscore the problem. Pete, as I observed him relating in that first interview with his mother and with me, was more anxious-oppositional than passive-effeminate. He seemed typical of this larger, acting-out group of adolescent boys, however, in that there was an additional specific training model for the acting-out itself. Mrs. Woodridge, like the mothers of the other boys in this group, misbehaved in similar ways, or expected acting-out behavior from Pete.

Adolescent boys in this oppositional group cover the anxieties related to felt inadequacies as boys by chronic aggressiveness. Usually they express this by oppositional patterns of a passive character—stubbornness, dawdling, plain negativism—

although sometimes they are actively aggressive. They drive dangerously fast on country roads, fight with other boys, and engage in spree drinking or drug experimentation coupled with stories of personal aggressive prowess. At other times they appear to be conforming, but they continually provoke adults or younger children in their own families. By the use of procrastination and other negative measures, they covertly show their underlying aggressiveness. When these oppositional tendencies invade the learning process, difficulties arise from their failing to hear directions, to follow through and complete tasks, or to relate with the external authority of the teacher and principal. Many gradually drop out of junior high or early senior high school, loaf around town, or in time run or simply drift away from their local communities. Some are aggressive enough to get into difficulty with local laws, so that they are committed to the child welfare agency and sent to residential treatment institutions or group work-camp facilities. There, through guidance counseling, training in real-work programs, and supervised peer relationships, many of these adolescent boys improve. Their identity problems, basic to their previous misbehavior and failure to learn, have been somewhat resolved.

But, because of the tendencies just described and the deeply entrenched conflicts in both Mrs. Woodridge and Pete, I was not at all optimistic about progress with them as our initial joint interview ended. Both seemed relatively unmodifiable at that point. Nonetheless, I set another appointment with them three days later.

My suspicions were borne out when, the day following our first interview, Mrs. Woodridge called in angry tears. She asked to see me at once. In an emergency interview with her that afternoon I learned that she had Pete jailed earlier that day when, in response to his mother's provocation, he had slashed the sofa with a knife and clouted her with a poker. In the face of this new crisis, I recommended to Mrs. Woodridge that she voluntarily commit Pete to the Kentucky Department for Human Resources. She did so. From jail this commitment eventually led Pete into a nine-month period of work-camp participation and group counseling.

After he returned home, Pete asked to talk with me again in the office. His self-regard was much higher than it had been previously. He now thought of himself as a young man who could eventually learn a trade, marry, and raise a family. Though his mother was unchanged, Pete spoke of his new-found ability to withstand her criticism of him, to grow around her. He wished to return to school locally until his sixteenth birthday, when he planned to enroll in the regional vocational school's training program in carpentry. Pete attributed his new feelings about himself to his group work-camp experience: "I learned there that I was really worth something as a man, and that I am not the louse my mother always said I was."

As was the case with several other oppositional boys I have followed, Pete had made significant progress in settling some important identity questions for himself. His basic warmth as a person enabled him, in time, to relate well with men and other boys and to learn from them greater self-regard and better ways of handling himself as a growing young man.

The First Interview: What the Evaluator Must Do. First interviews with crisis-stricken families vary widely in both focus and direction, depending on the nature of the emotional crisis itself. But in most cases the parent who calls emphasizes problems in the child or adolescent, designating him or her as the patient, rather than the whole family. The investigator, however, must consider three possibilities.

(1) Obviously, there may indeed be internal problems in the child that contribute significantly to the school phobia, drug abuse, delinquency, sexual promiscuity, running away, or other behavior that has brought the family to a crisis point.

(2) Often, however, the way the family relates together and communicates aggravates minor difficulties in the children, who then present the aberrant behavior being labeled as a problem by the parent who calls for help.

(3) A combination of family factors and internal problems in the child may be interacting to produce the emotional crisis.

The evaluator must attempt to sort out and clarify these various internal (that is within the child) and family factors in his first interview with the family.

As stated earlier in this chapter, the evaluator can frequently learn a great deal from the views of the family's functioning offered by a sibling older than the designated patient. An older sibling may well not be involved centrally, or immediately, in the crisis itself; often he is closer to the periphery. This position, reinforced by his having observed the younger sibling's growth throughout his life and by his observations of the family's functioning now and in the past, enables him to make more accurate comments about family members than either his troubled parents or his younger brother or sister. Embroiled together in crisis, the parents and the child they designate as the patient are frequently too emotionally involved to see the overall situation with much objectivity.

As a rule, I explain the value of including an older sibling in the first interview at the time of the parent's inquiry, and I put it in much the same terms as outlined here. Although I make it a matter of choice, I generally underscore the sibling's value sufficiently so that most families do, indeed, bring him along. Siblings younger than the designated patient can be included as well in the initial, joint family interview if the evaluator judges, during the parent's call, that these younger children are involved significantly in the situation. But if they are peripheral to the crisis, I generally exclude them, at least initially, in favor of an older sibling's inclusion. Of course, sometimes there is no older sibling available, and the evaluator has no choice but to interview jointly the principal family members in the crisis.

Where possible, the evaluator should ensure that the appropriate sibling is included in the first interview.

The First Interview: The Sibling's Importance Demonstrated. One family I saw pointed up the value of including an older sibling as an observer of family functioning. The father, dean of a large division of a local university, called me one afternoon in much anxiety about his seventeen-year-old son, Brent. With a rush of words this man told me over the telephone that mumps encephalitis had left Brent moderately mentally retarded and somewhat neurologically handicapped since the age of three. The boy, the father indicated, had needed much sheltering love and care all along. They had given this, he said, and Brent responded well by being a dutiful, compliant, obedient—and dependent—child. He had learned academic skills to about a fourth-grade level during his years in classes for educable mentally retarded children. Even Brent's early adolescence had not presented insurmountable problems to the family as a whole, the father continued.

But, over the past six months, he and his wife had been continually upset over Brent's angrily stubborn, defiant behavior. This behavior was completely new for him. A crisis had been precipitated the day before the father called me. Brent had demanded of his mother that he be given driving lessons. The mother had tried to explain that his neurological handicap militated against this. In a rage the boy had slapped his mother, then run from the house, discharging a shotgun of his father's (taken forcibly from a locked gun cabinet in the den) against the side of the family's new car. The mother had then called a neighbor to take the now-empty weapon from her son. Both the mother and Brent had apparently been frightened and anxious following this event. Together, that evening, the parents had decided to seek help. On the advice of their family physician, the father decided to call me that following afternoon. He agreed to come in with his wife, Brent, and their nineteen-year-old daughter Susan to a joint interview set for early the following morning.

As we sat down together in the office, I explained to the family the two goals that an evaluator has in this kind of interview:

(1) To help the family clarify the factors that played a part in producing the recent crisis.

(2) To make plans, together with the family, that might produce better, more adaptive functioning on the part of all family members in the future.

Then, addressing myself directly to Susan, I explained that I really needed her views of the family to assist me in these first two interview goals—that I saw her role in the interview as a partner with me in observing the family's functioning. She understood this part she was to play, she indicated, but then did not speak for the next half-hour. During that time, the parents' own anxieties intervened. They retraced the story of the crisis, the outline of which the father had given me over the telephone a day earlier. As they did this, I was impressed with several points about the couple. They were genuinely fond of Brent and seemed to have done much to nurture him throughout his growth. Furthermore, both parents seemed to me quiet, polite, almost reserved people beneath their immediate anxiety. But they were upset over and did not understand this new, angry, defiant behavior in Brent. And they clearly stated they felt at a complete loss as to how to cope with it.

While his parents talked, Brent himself sat saying nothing. A muscular, well-dressed, rather handsome youth, he showed the neurological stigmata the father had referred to in the form of cerebral-palsied movements of his right upper extremity and neck and the language deficits commensurate with his intellectual retardation. Brent felt guilty, or "bad inside," as I helped him to reflect on his feelings about the crisis situation. Then his eyes flashed and anger edged his voice as he told me his parents babied him all the time and prohibited activities he wanted to do, like driving a car. The mother then spoke. In a weak, helpless way she said she knew Brent wanted to do things other seventeen-year-olds did, but there were so many problems he had that prevented this. She stopped talking abruptly, and began to cry. Her husband at once spoke consolingly to her.

At just this point Susan, slowly at first, but then more boldly with my encouragement to continue, spoke up. "Dr. Looff, in one way Brent's right to be angry so often this past year. He's grown, and he's very sensitive about the differences between himself and other kids. He knows he doesn't do as well as others in schoolwork, and his palsy handicap makes it hard for him to do other things, since he's righthanded and the problem is on that side. But he wants to do the things others do, I know. And he suffers because he can't." She said she had seen him look longingly at boys playing basketball in the neighbors' backyard, and had seen him get angry when his homework came hard for him, as it normally did. She revealed that she understood her parents' protective feelings about Brent, but that she felt "it doesn't help him when the folks try to cover it all up. I mean, they try to smooth over what Brent is feeling. I think they deny he gets so mixed up inside, or that he is growing up. They end up treating him like they've always done, as a younger child. But Dr. Looff, how can my brother really take pride in himself unless he's trained properly as a grown person? I think he's outgrown those special classes of his. Shouldn't he be taught some kind of trade now?

There must be something he can do he would like. And there's just one more thing I can say. And please, Mom and Dad, don't get me wrong here, either. It's just that I don't feel my folks can handle Brent anymore, Dr. Looff. It was okay as long as he was younger, and quiet like he was. But he's big now, and he's upset much of the time, and angry. And all that is too hard for them to take." She suggested that there ought to be some way for Brent to live apart from them, with other boys his age who had the same problems, and get the training he needed.

There was silence in the room for a moment after Susan stopped talking. Then, with tears in his eyes, the father said he really, "deep down," agreed with everything she had said. He mentioned that he and his wife loved Brent dearly, that they had sensed for some time that he needed vocational training and felt that his present school program was not heading in this direction, but that the thought of sending him away made him feel guilty and anxious. He also agreed that Susan was correct in seeing much of Brent's current defiant behavior as the result of underlying anxious-depressed feelings. "As Susan says, how can Brent feel good about himself when he's not into the same things other boys his age are. I'd be depressed and unhappy, too, I guess."

It seemed that Susan's summary had given her father permission, as it were, to feel and speak similarly—to validate her views of the family's functioning. That interview, and several succeeding ones with the entire family, built upon this beginning consensual validation of family relationships and feelings. In time, a plan was worked out whereby Brent was enrolled in a private residential treatment and vocational training school for neurologically handicapped youths. As Susan herself had predicted in her earliest summary of her family, this plan met everyone's needs much more appropriately than any other might have done.

The Family in Succeeding Interviews. As with the foregoing family case example, most families in crisis do best, I've found, if kept together in succeeding interviews. The same twofold aim continues, building on the first interview: to understand and resolve the crisis, and to plan interim and long-term goals for the family and its individual members. This seems to be valid because crises so often depend primarily upon disturbed interpersonal relationships among family members, rather than upon problems individual members may have.

In the family just described there were, obviously, both interpersonal and individual problems. But, even in this instance, planning for Brent's individual needs proceeded best from a whole-family interview position. Only after they clarified the family crisis in terms of relationships and feelings, with Susan's summary leading the way, were they in an emotional position to see Brent's own needs in perspective, and only then could they be helped to plan appropriately for the boy.

In the next chapter we return to considering the differential diagnostic evaluation of children whose families are not in crisis, even though the parents are concerned about the individual learning and behavior problems their children are having.

Chapter 5.

Meeting the Young Child: His First Interview

Establishing a Relationship. The interviewer's first task begins the moment the child crosses the threshold of the waiting room for his first interview—namely, the task of creating a favorable emotional setting within which he and the child can relate and interact. The youngster must feel sufficiently at ease to express his needs and concerns. Much of this chapter is devoted to a discussion of specific techniques for the interviewer, techniques that aid what I call the forward flow of the interview. The same methods can often facilitate succeeding interviews as well.

But these interview techniques, description and examples of which make up the bulk of this chapter, are clearly secondary in importance to laying the groundwork of a good relationship between the interviewer and the child himself. Some key facts about child development make this so. The preschool and the school-age child are still quite dependent upon significant adults in their lives for approval, support, discipline, and direction. Although the older school-age child is more peer-oriented, and depends somewhat less on relationships with adults for guidance and support than the preschool child, he nonetheless requires adult direction in order to meet and master new experiences. Obviously the evaluation, and the evaluator himself, represent for the child a new experience with a new adult—who at first is bound to be strange. Thus, within that first interview, especially at the very beginning, all the child's feelings about this experience with this new person naturally are uppermost. And many of these feelings are dysphoric, or negative. The child may inwardly feel varying degrees of anxiety, doubt, anger, shame, disappointment, and sadness. In his past relationships with adults—assuming that some of them, at least, have been supportive for him—the young child has turned to them to help him with such troublesome feelings. The interviewer, realizing that the young child will probably turn to him as well, can utilize this tendency to assist the child in several ways in these first interviews.

At the very outset, children are not apt to talk spontaneously about their inner negative feelings. But, troubled and generally silent at first, they do depend on us, as adults who have been made significant by their parents' choice, for guidance and direction in this new experience and for some help with their troubled feelings. This dependence on the evaluator makes the child, at that first meeting, very sensitive to the evaluator's own feeling state, to the words he uses to outline and direct the interview experience, and to his natural ways of relating with the young child himself. If the evaluator is reasonably comfortable (not unduly anxious) at the beginning of a first interview with a young child, if he is willing to say some things at the beginning of the interview that map out the direction in which the two of them will go, and if he brings to the interview some warmth and friendliness and some degree of liking for children, all this is readily apparent to the child. Perceiving these qualities in this new, still strange adult, the child immediately receives some aid in meeting and mastering his feelings about the interview experience itself. So aided, many children can then proceed to share some of their thoughts and feelings about themselves with the interviewer, who—as they have just experienced—can be both understanding and supportive. Just what the evaluator can do and say at the very beginning of the initial interview to demonstrate his understanding and support is illustrated in the following discussion by the example of Charlie Russell's first interview with me. Following that example are descriptions of methods and techniques an interviewer can use (1) to begin to establish a relationship at the very beginning of which the young child can experience tangible emotional aid and support from the evaluator, and (2) to assist the child to begin to share his thoughts and feelings with him.

As the child and I meet and begin to relate, and once our talking has been set in forward motion, I steer that first interview toward getting the child's own story of events and feelings important to him over a wide range of his activities.

Together we attempt to gain some understanding of the child's many interpersonal relationships with parents, siblings, peers, other family members, teachers, and so on. As he discusses these, the story of his worries and problems often begins to emerge. I begin to get a picture of his conflicts and the ways in which he attempts to meet them.

Once a relationship is begun, the first interview thus becomes for many children a historical one. The focus of my second diagnostic interview is somewhat different. By the time of the second interview, the child has often been helped because our relating together has assuaged his troubled feelings about the evaluation experience, and he is thereby better prepared to go over certain special paper-and-pencil tests with me, to reveal himself somewhat further in various semiprojective fantasy items, to take a reading test for me, and to review certain aspects of his functioning that, raised initially in that broad first interview, need further clarification. How seven-year-old Charlie Russell and I got along in our first interview is the story we return to at this point in his evaluation.

As the Interview Develops. Alice Russell was the parent who brought Charlie to my office for his first interview. She had prepared him the night before for our appointment. Later she indicated that Charlie was unusually quiet as she picked him up from school that afternoon and while they were driving to the office. Charlie was slightly ahead of his mother as they came through the waiting-room door. A sturdy, well-developed lad with curly brown hair and large brown eyes, he stepped across the threshold somewhat hesitantly. A somewhat crooked grin slowly spread across his face as I came from my office to greet them. In his free hand he clutched some drawings. In the hesitation of his steps, and in the crooked quality of his smile, I felt that Charlie was showing the anxiety any seven-year-old might feel on meeting a strange doctor in a strange setting.

As they came in, I shook hands with Mrs. Russell, and then I turned and greeted Charlie with a handshake. "Well, you must be Charlie. I'm very pleased to meet you. You know, I had a chance to meet and talk with your folks the other day, but I didn't get to meet you until right now. I guess that sort of makes us strangers—for a while, anyway." Charlie's grin straightened out somewhat as he responded to this accurate reflection of the situation and his feelings. "Yeah, I never did see you before! But my Mom says you're pretty okay. I brought you some pictures from school." As I accepted them, I said, "Thank you, Charlie. There are probably some pretty good stories that go with these pictures. Maybe you can tell me the stories while we're talking together now, for an hour. Mrs. Russell, while Charlie and I are talking, drawing, and playing together this next hour in my playroom, what do you plan to do? Stay here and look at the magazines in the waiting room, or go get a cup of coffee at the restaurant around the corner? Charlie and I will be finished talking, so you can go home together, around ten minutes of four." Charlie, I could see, was watching me intently as I spoke, rounding out the situation for the three of us. Remarking that she had some shopping to do in the immediate area, Mrs. Russell said, "Go with Dr. Looff, Charlie. Mother will be back for you soon." She then turned and started out the waiting-room door. I said, "Let me show you where the playroom is, Charlie—where you and I will be while your mother's shopping." Although he was quiet, Charlie came readily with me into the large playroom. His face had a studied expression, but he was not near tears, nor did he protest his mother's leaving. In this way, I learned quite naturally that Charlie did not experience significant separation anxiety on leaving one of his parents. This fact corroborated a point the Russells had made earlier to me regarding Charlie's functioning quite well when left on his own.

As we came into the playroom, I said to Charlie, "I saved a special chair for you," as I indicated that I would like him to sit in a particular spot. Along one wall in my playroom is a low, eight-foot-long oak kindergarten table that makes an excellent table for talking across the corner, for drawing, for taking special paper-and-pencil tests, for games, for doll play, and the like. I generally sit at one end of the table in a kindergarten-size chair, while the child, if he isn't playing elsewhere in the room, sits across the corner of the table from me in a similar chair. This arrangement brings me to the young child's level for talking and drawing, provides comfortable seating, and positions the child with maximum work space in front of him. Charlie accepted this arrangement quite naturally, and began to spread his school drawings out as we talked further.

As we sat down, I commented to Charlie, "Your're getting to be a big fellow. Let's see, how old are you now—eight?" My "guessing" a year above his known age pleased the boy. "No, I'm seven," he replied with a grin. Clearly, the device had helped him a bit to feel less small and vulnerable in the still new, and therefore still stressful, situation of our meeting and beginning to relate with one another. "Well," I said, "I would have guessed you were older. When will you be eight?" Charlie stated his birthday, and went on to give his school, his teacher's name, the names of two friends in his class, his sister's name and age, and the fact that he had a rock collection that he had started after the family's summer vacation trip to New Mexico. By then he was settling into the relationship somewhat more comfortably.

"Charlie, I can see it doesn't take you long to start making a new friend. I'm getting the idea that you don't think I'm so strange, now." Grinning broadly, the boy nodded his assent. "And I can see you are a good talker, too. I'm glad of that. I'm wondering if your folks told you what kind of a doctor I am, and what I'm interested in?" Charlie replied that his mother had told him I was a worry-doctor. "And she said you don't give shots! Boy, am I glad of that! Doctor Thompson sure gives those to me sometimes! Elizabeth cries when she gets stuck. I don't cry, but I sure don't like it. That's funny— a worry-doctor!" He laughed, and I joined in. Then, as a way both of rounding out the situation for Charlie by defining our mutual roles in the interview and of reinforcing the talking-with-feeling capability the boy had already given evidence of possessing, I said, "Well, I can see your mother gave you the right idea about me. Yes, I'm a worry-doctor interested in the worries and problems all kids have growing up. And I'm interested in the fun things, too. You know, the things you think about and do that maybe don't have worries with them. But all kids have some worries. Your folks were here the other day, and they talked with me about you, Charlie, and about how they feel things are going in the family. They feel you may have some worries. So that's why they brought you here to talk with me. It looks like we're all working on a worry puzzle together." Here I drew a ring in the air with my finger, indicating different points on the ring as I talked about the role each one of us could play in figuring this whole matter out. "Your Mom and Dad have some ideas, like pieces in a puzzle. Then you have some ideas and feelings, too, Charlie. And that's another very important part of the puzzle we're all working on. Then I want to talk with your teacher in private sometime. She has some ideas about how you're doing in your work, and about how you get along with the other kids and with her. These are all parts of the puzzle, too. What do you think of my idea of a worry puzzle?"

Charlie listened intently while this somewhat lengthy definition of our mutual roles was being established. But, like many other bright, verbal, feeling-oriented school-age children, he picked up readily on the worry-puzzle analogy.

"I get worried when I get mad at Sissy. She won't play school with me, and I get mad and hit her!" Tears were coming into Charlie's eyes as he said this. I reflected that telling me about hitting his sister seemed to make him feel sad. Here, as at all future points in our two diagnostic interviews, a reflecting-his-feelings approach on my part reinforced the flow of Charlie's talking. He did not require play items, drawings, or games to open up communication. His behavior pointed up the axiom that talk, with feelings, speeds things up in many diagnostic interviews. Obviously, not all children are as verbal and as spontaneous about sharing their troubled feelings as was Charlie, and the development of first interviews with less talkative children is discussed later on in this chapter, as further case examples are cited. But the point remains that for many children like Charlie, feeling-oriented talking is natural and can rather quickly be achieved, and interviews proceed best if this capacity is utilized.

"I feel bad inside when I hit Sissy! But she won't play with me right. She's supposed to write down the spelling words I give her." I wondered aloud here to the boy: "What's your best guess about this, Charlie? Do you think Sissy is being plain stubborn and just won't write down what you tell her to? Or is it hard for her, because she's just four years old, to know how to spell all the big words you can in the second grade?" This "best guess" approach helped Charlie be reflective. "Well, maybe you're right. She is just four—that's what Mom says, too. Only she doesn't say it. She yells it at me! That's what worries me. If I get mad at Sissy, she runs and tells Mom. Then I catch it—oh, boy!" Charlie told me at this point that he was frequently spanked, sent to his room, or had television taken from him for an evening if he played rough with his sister. Reminding him that he had told me he felt "bad inside" when he lost his temper and struck Elizabeth, I speculated again: "Since you feel so bad when you hit Sissy because she can't write all the big words, what about playing school with someone who maybe can spell as well as you do? You know, someone like a friend in the neighborhood." Charlie looked crestfallen. Just as anxiety of high intensity will frequently disrupt play activities of a young child in an interview, so, too, can anxiety disrupt the flow of talk. I said, "Uh, oh! Charlie, it looks like I've asked about something here that makes you unhappy and stop talking. You seem to figure other things out pretty well. Maybe you can turn on another best guess and figure out what made you upset just now." Tears came to the boy's eyes again. "It's those other kids. They don't like me at all! All they ever do is run away or tease me!" In spite of my gentle but firm probing in this area of his relationships with his peers, Charlie was not able just then to make the connection his parents had surmised, namely, that he used his intelligence to take over a group, to be bossy, to demand that he be the leader and planner of the group's activities. As a result, the Russells had indicated to me earlier, children his own age shunned Charlie, or teased him for his temper tantrums. He was left, accordingly, to play the ringleader with a small neighborhood group of preschool children who docilely followed his whims.

Charlie was, however, able to make a connection, with my leading and support, between his quick display of temper with his sister and his school problems. I asked him, "Well, it seems like you do kind of lose your temper with Sissy when she makes you angry. I wonder, Charlie—since we're still working on this puzzle together—if anything like this ever happens in school. What do you think?" Reflecting a moment, Charlie replied: "That Mrs. Snyder is about as dumb as Sissy! All those dumb baby words she gives us! And those dumb problems. Anybody can do those!" At this point, I wondered about how he did in reading. "Oh, that's my best thing. I can read my Dad's encyclopedias pretty good. There are some of the words I get mixed up on, but he helps me. That's where

I get all my stuff about rocks and dinosaurs." Charlie then launched into a long dissertation on paleontology. From his vocabulary level, from his general fund of such information, and from the rich, colorful, abstract way in which he joined words and concepts together, I made the informal clinical assessment that his verbal skills placed him in the high bright normal to superior range of intellectual functioning.

His discourse over, I led him back to his feelings that Mrs. Snyder gave him "dumb things to do." "Yeah, who wants to do any of that! I sure don't! I had that stuff at home, in kindergarten." Because he was aware of strong negative feelings toward work in the classroom that probably was beneath his skills, I sought further clarification of Charlie's functioning at school by commenting, "Sometimes, when kids are bright, like you are, they get impatient with what they feel are baby, dumb things in school. Maybe they sometimes get so impatient, or even mad, they won't finish their regular work. Or they get so mad they lose patience and do something like mischief in the room." Charlie ruefully grinned as a way, I felt, of consensually validating my speculation. "Sure, I get impatient," he said. "Wouldn't you?" He did not particularly like my confronting him just then, gently but firmly, with my understanding—gained from his folks, who "love you, and were telling me how things go in school with you sometimes because they want to help you"—that he often did not complete assignments or acted up in an angry way in the classroom. However, he agreed this was often true, even though he did not like the confrontation.

Summarizing to this point, I said: "Charlie, let me see if I'm getting a clear pricture of what's happening with you. You're bright, and you sometimes feel mad because Sissy won't play school like you can, or because the teacher gives you only dumb baby work. You get so mad sometimes you lose your temper and hit Sissy, or the other kids, or make some other kind of mischief." Charlie indicated, somewhat ruefully, that I was getting the picture quite clearly indeed.

At this juncture, since we had established some important conflictual themes, I felt the interview should be steered toward pleasanter topics. Charlie needed the pressure off him for a few minutes, and I needed to know if there were, indeed, less emotionally charged areas of his functioning.

Grinning from ear to ear, Charlie role-played a fun-filled football game with his father in response to my statement: "You know, Charlie, all boys have some fun times and some tough times with their dads. How about you and your dad. How do you two get along?" "He teaches me all about football, basketball, and baseball. Sometimes he takes a whole Saturday off just to teach me and we play together. I really do like that!" The only "tough times" Charlie alluded to were spankings received from his father when he struck his sister or his dog. To similar questions about his relationship with his mother, Charlie replied that she "is a real pretty lady who cooks my favorite—spaghetti and meatballs. Sometimes she yells at me, like I told you. But sometimes, when she gets mad, she says no, I can't have something. Then I wait and butter her up!" A few further questions on my part drew from Charlie that he meant his mother's "no" was frequently a "maybe" that might become a "yes." He seemed to be corroborating his mother's vacillating, inconsistent ways of correcting him, which both of his parents had mentioned.

We moved on to questions about his hobbies, special interests, talents, favorite play themes, and the like. His replies indicated that rocks and dinosaurs were his special reading interests, and that reading itself was a frequent pastime, but not his only one. He had a personal ambition, he said, to be an archeologist when he grew up. He correctly defined the kinds of activities a man like this would engage in. His interests in bows and arrows, dart guns, B-B guns, flying kites, team sports, and games like his favorite erector set suggested to me that Charlie had a healthy interest in competitive games and play materials.

Near the end of that first interview hour Charlie indicated that he wanted me to take note of the pencil drawings he had brought in with him and unfolded on the work table as we sat talking together. He selected one of the drawings for comment. "I call it my watered-down picture. 'Watered-down' is the title." (See illustration.) Examining the picture carefully, I told Charlie, "Yeah, there must be a really good story that goes with this picture." He sketched in several associations to his drawing. "There's this boy dragon—you see, the one snorting fire out of his nostrils. He's pulling that man, the fire marshal, like crazy in that fire engine! The fireman made a stupid

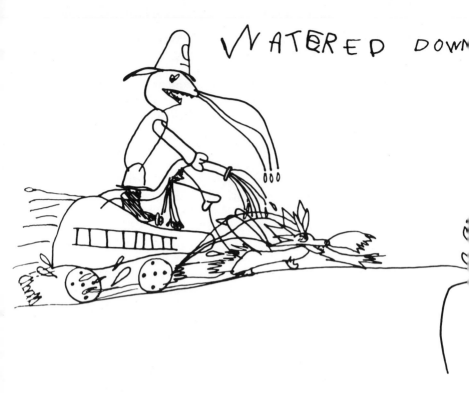

WATERED DOWN

mistake! He decided to save the fire department some money by having a dragon pull the engine instead of spending money on gas, but he didn't realize he was getting a powerful boy dragon who went too fast. They're about to go over the cliff! The dragon just wanted to see the flower growing there, but he got going so fast he can't stop himself. So the fireman's trying to water him down to slow him up!" I told Charlie he had drawn a wonderful picture and told me a wonderful story because I thought it was "pretty much like it happens with you." And then I went over his story with him, substituting his intellectual interests for the flower, himself for the boy dragon who sometimes gets impatient and can't stop himself in his interests or his anger, and his parents and his teacher for the fireman trying to stop him when he cannot stop himself.

The interview ended with my summary that I saw Charlie as a fine boy. "You have good stuffings in you, Charlie," I told him. "You like the things all boys your age do. And you're bright—you've got good brain power. But you've got a problem with handling your anger sometimes. You get mad and impatient and pop off at people. But that messes it up for you, too. And you feel bad inside, you've told me, once that happens. Maybe in the next five days, before I see you again for your next visit, Charlie, you could practice on your patience a bit. It's all right for you to get angry—we all do. But it's not okay for any one of us to hit. So maybe you could slow yourself down—you know, sort of water yourself down—if Sissy makes you mad and you need to stop yourself before you both end up over the cliff. I wonder, what do you think of all this?"

Charlie agreed that the summary was accurate. He enlarged on it by saying, "You're right—I need more patience. Maybe when Sissy makes me mad I could count to ten so I won't hit her. No, that wouldn't work—I'd better take time to count to a million!" We both laughed. Then I said, "Fine, maybe something like this million-thing can help you put the brakes on your anger—help you to be patient enough not to hit her in anger. And remember, we all get angry sometimes. That's okay. But we can find safe ways of being angry. Words don't hurt, but hits do. So I like your idea of counting to get patience. Practice that, and see what you think of my idea of telling Sissy you're angry with safe, angry words." We agreed to talk some more about "patience and school papers" at our next interview. Charlie then left his one drawing with me as a gift. He was grinning and waving back at me as he went out of the office.

FACTORS AIDING THE FLOW OF THE INTERVIEW
WITH THE YOUNG CHILD

From young children like Charlie, I have through the years learned some important considerations about one's first interviews with them. These children have taught me that there are certain factors which definitely aid the flow, or forward motion, of these initial interviews. Once set in motion, an interview tends to have a definite momentum of its own. The crucial matter for the interviewer, then, is to facilitate its beginning. As one of my former trainees put it: "These factors aiding the flow of the interview Dr. Looff talks about might better be called a 'shove in the right direction.'" For ease in examining each of these somewhat distinct but certainly interrelated factors, they are listed here separately.

(1) *The interviewer can anticipate how the young child will relate with him.* Before he sees the child for the first time, the evaluator has interviewed the parents himself or familiarized himself with the information already obtained by other professional colleagues. Thus, he has knowledge of the nature and history of the presenting problems and the emotional climate of the home, and—of crucial importance—he has some understanding of how the child relates with others. This briefing provides the evaluator with working hypotheses about the child's difficulties and gives him some expectation of what he will find in his diagnostic interviews. He has some advance knowledge of the way the child will relate to him as a new adult in a new and therefore stressful situation. In Charlie's case, his parents had in their initial joint interview told me Charlie was a friendly, outgoing lad who "never knew a stranger" and enjoyed the company of adults. Therefore, I could anticipate that his anxiety on meeting me would be minimal, that he could in all probability separate easily from the parent who brought him, and that he would settle into the interview quickly and comfortably. In effect, then, the evaluator generally finds that the shape or quality of their initial relationship is like those the child has been reported to have with other adults.

(2) *The evaluation (and supportive treatment) of the child begins in the waiting room as the interviewer rounds out the situation for him.* Earlier I mentioned the necessity of creating a favorable emotional setting for the interviews, a task that begins as soon as the child first enters the waiting room. It is precisely at this moment that the child shows us his anticipatory anxiety as well as the emotional level at which he functions—how he tends to cope with new stresses. The reader will recall that Charlie showed some concerns through the slight hesitancy of his steps and through the somewhat crooked quality of the grin that began to spread over his face as he met me. The interviewer has an opportunity, right there during

those first minutes in the waiting room, to put the child's anxiety (shown nonverbally) into words and to state it in such a way that the child will not feel he has been dealt a blow. One way the interviewer can divest his feeling-oriented statement of any such harsh impact is to share in the child's feeling position. I put Charlie's anxiety, shown nonverbally, into words that didn't make him feel like the only bug on the pin: "... but I didn't get to meet you until right now. I guess that sort of makes *us strangers*—for a while, anyway."

The interviewer has other important ways of rounding out the situation for the child within the first few minutes of their meeting besides helping the child put his anticipatory anxiety into words. "Rounding out" the interview situation includes all the things the interviewer can do to structure, define, and clarify the experience for the child. As the young child enters the interview, there are many unfamiliar elements about this new experience. Most children have some fear of the unknown, but their anxiety can be lessened if the interviewer familiarizes them with what is coming and thus rounds out the situation for them. Most children can cope with an experience better if at least the outline of it is made known to them. That is the purpose of statements like the ones I made to Charlie and Mrs. Russell as I met them in the waiting room and as Charlie and I moved together to the playroom. I mentioned our respective role definitions (I was a "worry-doctor" and we would be working on a "worry puzzle" together); the length of the interview and where his mother would pass the time were clearly defined; and all my introductory statements to Charlie oriented him toward talking about his feelings as a means of further defining the interview experience. The interviewer can further round out the situation by showing the young child where the bathroom is and by commenting pleasantly on something familiar and tangible ("That's a nice green shirt you're wearing, Charlie"). After an introduction along these lines most children, like Charlie, can separate easily and begin relating and talking with the interviewer in the playroom.

Many children, however, are much more fearful and inhibited than Charlie was on meeting me. The ease or difficulty with which the child can separate from his parents to go with the interviewer to the playroom is often extremely revealing both of the child-parent relationship and of the child's degree of differentiation from his mother and father. The child or the parents may suffer from marked separation anxiety, and it is well in that case to allow all of them to go in together to the playroom for at least a few minutes. In such instances, the interviewer makes a rapid assessment of the family's emotional functioning while everyone is in the waiting room and plans accordingly. Then he puts his observations into words.

For example, a young couple, both of whom were physicians in their early thirties, sought my help for their five-year-old daughter Beth. Beth's chief concerns, from what they told me earlier, seemed to involve separation anxiety. The family had moved each year since the child was born. Each move was unsettling to the couple, particularly to the mother, who had a tendency to overreact anxiously to stress of any type by becoming angry and nongiving to her husband and their child. The presenting problems in Beth were school fears. She separated from her parents to attend school but cried throughout most of each kindergarten morning, had frequent nightmares, clung to them on shopping trips, and sucked her thumb. From their story, I anticipated that Beth would have difficulty leaving her mother to go with me to the playroom.

At the appointed hour, I could hear Beth crying loudly "I don't want to!" out in the hallway. Her mother led her gently but firmly into my waiting room and sat down in a chair near the door. As I greeted them, Beth crawled into her mother's lap, buried her face in her mother's shoulder, clung tightly, and sobbed loudly, "I don't want to go! Please don't make me go!" At this point I said, "Gee, it looks like you're feeling very unhappy right now, Beth. You know, lots of girls and boys feel just like you do when they meet a strange doctor for the very first time. I guess your mother told you I am a different kind of children's doctor than she is [the mother is a pediatrician]. She looks in kids' ears, and down their mouths, and listens to their chests. But I don't do that. No, I'm a worry-doctor." Finger in her mouth, Beth was half looking at me from her mother's shoulder at this point. "That doesn't mean that I try to make kids worried. I'm just interested in the worries all girls and boys have growing up. One of your worries right now, I guess, is that mother will leave you. I can understand that. Lots of girls feel that way sometimes. So why don't we have mother come on in with us to my playroom until we get to know each other better. You know, until we won't be strangers anymore."

At this verbal signal Beth's mother put the child down and, following me, led her into the playroom. I sat in my usual kindergarten-size chair at one end of the work table. Her mother seated Beth on the chair across the corner of the table from me and knelt down beside her. I repeated what I had said in the waiting room. Then I added comments about the pretty dress that Beth was wearing, and said that I guessed, since she was getting so big, she was six. "No," she said, taking her finger from her mouth and moving her folded arm from her tear-soaked face so that she could see me, "I'm five." She spread her fingers, like a fan. "Hey, that's good, Beth!" I said. "I guess you're learning to count." "My Mommy teaches me. Mikey [her three-year-old brother, in nursery school] goes to school, too. He's all alone." More tears. "I guess, Beth, it makes you sad and unhappy when your family isn't all in one place. Lots of girls feel like that, sometimes." Beth and I were then able to exchange brief, identifying comments about her school, her teacher, where she lived, who lived there, and her dog Diane.

I told her a funny story about my own dog, Charlie, a setter, who brings home things like baseball gloves, leashes, and even a toy rubber duck from his wanderings in the park across from our house. Beth unplugged her mouth and grinned wetly. Next I said, "You know what? You look like the kind of girl who would know what a Hoo-Heimer is!" She didn't know, it turned out, but she listened intently as I described the Dr. Seuss birthday book story about Hoo-Heimers, those mythical animals that carry in the birthday presents on their backs. Again she unplugged her mouth, and this time she laughed faintly. "I saw a green Hoo-Heimer once," she said. "Wonderful," I replied, "You were lucky! Most of them are yellow. You just don't get to see green ones very often!" Beth then began, somewhat anxiously, to rattle on to me oblivious of her mother who, still kneeling at the child's side through these five minutes, began to question with her eyebrows whether it was now time for her to leave the playroom. I said, "Beth, I think you're starting to feel better. You're finding out that I don't have two heads and breathe fire like a dragon." Beth laughed. "Since I'm not a dragon, but just want to talk with you some more like we're starting to, I think maybe we could stay here together, talking like this, while we send mother to the room just out there. And we'll leave the door open."

The mother rose to her feet, stated she would be just outside, and left the playroom. As she was leaving, I asked Beth (who did not protest the separation at this point, nor did she leave her chair), "I guess you know what happens when you and I finish talking in here today?" Beth shrugged. "You go home!" She smiled wanly.

I had learned anew from this experience a fact of cardinal importance: If the child and the parents are helped to tolerate their anxiety, this obvious respect for their separation fears will prove an important step in their being able to overcome them. What made Beth's separation anxiety gradually tolerable for her that morning was a combination of several factors—her mother's being allowed to be with her for a few more minutes; my being friendly; my reflecting her feelings; my telling tales that reinforced what she was beginning to say on her own (the dog stories, for example); and my stating, in effect, that the planned separation from her mother was for a limited period only: "I guess you know what happens when we finish talking—you go home!" I call this latter technique "putting a period at the end of the sentence." It rounds out, or shapes definitively, the situation for the child with such separation fears. Fearful children can often cope with a situation that has been thus defined as self-limited. The bit about Hoo-Heimers was designed to tap her five-year-old capacity for fantasy, in a way that would make her laugh. Laughter alleviates many moments of pain for children in their interviews, and it helped make the interview situation more tolerable for Beth that morning. We related better as a result.

(3) *Talk speeds things up in a diagnostic interview. The interviewer should also go after feelings and keep reflecting these back to the child.* Such statements as the ones I made initially to Charlie and to Beth in the waiting room, in addition to their therapeutic function of alleviating anxiety, also present a model for all further transactions between the interviewer and the child. That model is a feeling-oriented, talking one. As they begin to relate together, both the interviewer and the child learn to put feelings into words. They learn to label accurately feelings caused by situations and events in the

child's life. Such clarification, or consensual validation, of events and feelings can be an important therapeutic accompaniment of any diagnostic interview. Children, as would adults, generally experience a rapid rise in self-esteem when they have been praised by the interviewer for talking along with him and for gradually putting events and feelings into words. Such praise is a powerful social reinforcer, prompting the child to talk further. Thus it aids the forward flow of the interview. Charlie grinned when I said, "And I can see you're a good talker, too. I'm glad of that. You told me your feelings about your friends. You figured that out pretty good. So, I wonder, maybe you can begin to figure out how you feel about your sister." In response to that form of praise about talking with feeling, Charlie went on to relate more about himself.

(4) *Another technique the interviewer can use to encourage the sometimes hesitant child to talk about himself is "pump-priming."* The analogy here is to a long-idle hand-operated pump. With disuse, the leather lifters on the pump plunger dry out, and one cannot draw water. As a boy, I occasionally had to prime my grandmother's well pump by pouring in a little water from a pail to get it going. So the interviewer, faced with a hesitant child, often helps him begin talking by telling short stories about the kinds of problems other boys and girls have had who have come here, and by asking him gently if the stories fit his situation and feelings. If they don't, the child is encouraged to say how matters are different for him. Then, as he begins to talk, he is rewarded for so doing. ("Good for you, Sam. Now I see what you mean. You told me what happened—and how you felt.")

(5) *Universalization-generalization comments made by the interviewer are another effective means of helping the child talk more about himself.* If the child hears from the interviewer such comments as "All children have worries and problems growing up," he is not so apt to view himself as the only boy who was ever sad or lonely or angry. Universalization is the interviewer's way of keeping his inquiries from falling like blows: "Gee, Charlie, lots of boys would have some pretty tough feelings right after they hit their sisters. I wonder what your feelings were like?" Charlie, in that instance, went on to tell me he "felt bad [guilty] inside." As they grow and develop, children are sensitive to their mistakes and failures. Universal-

ization takes the sting out of the interviewer's attempts to talk over these troublesome events and feelings with the child. Sometimes the child is relieved to learn that the interviewer himself can share similar troublesome feelings—that universalization extends to him as well. "Kids can be cruel sometimes. I can remember how sad I felt inside when kids teased me sometimes in school. I wonder if kids have teased you, and how you felt?" To ask an already hesitant child directly, "Do kids tease you in school sometimes?" might hurt him, making him resistive to the point of not talking in the interview in any real depth.

(6) *In asking about the child's feelings, the interviewer avoids, if he can, labeling these feelings too early.* If he can be helped to say accurately how he felt in an event he is describing, the child will show us that he can be a good observer of his own functioning. We need to know whether he has this capacity. Therefore, the interviewer uses general terms that suggest feeling-content as he inquires about an event in the child's life, and he avoids too early use of specific feeling terms. "You know, Sam, all boys have both fun times and tough times with their dads. I wonder if you could tell me about some tough times you've had with your dad." The word "tough" here is a general term covering all types of negative, dysphoric feelings that children can experience. Its use encourages the child to think about negative feelings in a particular relationship or event but leaves him free, if he is able to do so, to say what particular type of negative feeling he experienced (sadness, anger, disappointment, discouragement, fear, loneliness).

If a child, however, does not have the capacity at first to accurately label specific kinds of positive and negative feelings he experiences, the interviewer supplies a list of these feelings and asks the child to choose among them. "Sam, all boys have tough times, sometimes, with their dads. Let's see, you told me your dad promised to take you fishing last Saturday but then something happened and he couldn't go. So then you couldn't go. But I'm not sure how all that made you feel. Some boys would feel disappointed, or sad, or angry, or lonely if that happened. You know, they would have different kinds of feelings. What were your feelings, I wonder?" Sam, in that instance, picked disappointment. Such an approach may help train the child to begin to observe more accurately the feeling-content of his own relationships and experiences and, again with the interviewer's constant encouragement and support, to talk about these.

(7) *The interviewer can use best-guess approaches to help the child observe his own functioning.* Some children are highly accurate observers, at times, of their own functioning. Others are not, or may show the capacity to clarify some events well and others poorly. In this instance, one technique is to recall for the child how well he observed himself and his feelings in one event, and to wonder aloud whether he can try a "best guess" approach to attempt to clarify the particular event under discussion, some aspects of which remain obscure for them both. "Charlie, you figured out real well that you feel bad inside when you hit Sissy. Now, since we both know you can figure out some things real well, I wonder if you can give me your best guess about how you feel inside when your teacher writes a note telling your folks that you haven't been turning in your school papers. You told me that she does that sometimes. But I'm still not sure how you feel when she does that. What's your best guess?" Charlie, in that instance, went on to say he guessed he felt both "bad inside, like when I hit Sissy, but I'm scared, too—Dad may spank me!" The interviewer praises the child—a verbal reward—when he makes a best guess. By this approach, obscure events are not seen as insurmountable obstacles in the interview, but rather as challenges the child may take on with the interviewer's support. If he figures out one area well, we tell him so. He is thereby encouraged to figure out something else. No matter how emotionally troubled the child may be, as a growing, developing person he looks for approval from the adults around him. When we praise him for his good observations about himself, we tap this natural desire and turn it to our mutual advantage in an interview.

(8) *The continual use of summary statements by the interviewer as the interview proceeds is another technique for aiding its forward flow.* As the child begins to reveal himself, summarizing aloud what he has been saying is frequently helpful. First of all, it shows that the interviewer is listening carefully to what the child has to say, which encourages him to talk further. The child feels supported because these

summaries indicate tangibly that the interviewer wants to understand him in his situation. Feeling supported, the child may reveal himself even more. Secondly, the summaries simultaneously provide reinforcement of the child's growing ability to observe his own functioning and give him an opportunity to change, or clarify, some part of his story. Obviously, the first telling of any event may not get all the facts and feelings straight. A summary by the interviewer may, then, be a half-story. The child hears it and is thereby encouraged to round out the remaining half of the tale. Charlie, at the end of one of my summaries, corrected me (and clarified the story for himself, too, in the process): "No, Dr. Looff, that's not right. I didn't say I hit my dog because I was mad at him. I mean I hit him because he runs away from me and I can't tie him up. Those big dogs around our house could tear Snoopy up in a fight. That scares me! So I try to tie him up." My prompt, corrected summary in response was: "Oh, now I see. You are saying you hit Sissy because you are mad at her. But you hit Snoopy because you are scared he will run off and be hurt in a dogfight." The summary device, at that time, had led to Charlie's being able to clarify for me, and for himself, that he had two different sets of feelings prompting the same aggressive personal behavior. That differentiation was essential before, in succeeding interviews, he could see the rationale behind my suggestions of better ways to cope with the events leading up to the two kinds of feelings.

(9) *The interviewer avoids overidentifying with the child.* Some children have an often uncanny way of attempting to maneuver us into a feeling position in which we side with them against parents and teachers. Although we would like to side-step the issue, we have all at times been manipulated into taking a stand somewhat against the parents. Issues like bedtimes, treats, and chores evoke the child's explicit efforts to have us brand his parents as unfair or worse. Obviously, no one wants to fall into this trap. Our best course of action, as persons engaged in diagnostic interviews with children, is rather to deflect the attempt by saying something like: "Well, I hear you feel a nine o'clock bedtime is unfair, Sam. But every family has its own ground rules. We have them, too, at our house, where I'm a dad and Mrs. Looff is a mother. Right now, though, I'm trying to get a clear picture of how you and

your dad and mother get along together. And how you feel. I hope that, by taking time to get this picture clear, we can all work on the worry puzzle together, so things go better for all of you in your family. Maybe we will find out that some things are unfair for you. Or we may find out that some things are unfair for your folks, too. If we do, I can talk with them, and with you, to see if all of you would be willing to try another way of getting along."

Such a comment leaves the child with the distinct feeling that his ideas and feelings are listened to, as well as those of his parents. He also hears that we as evaluators still see the parents as being in charge at home—we respect their authority position. This kind of comment further indicates that later on there may need to be some discussion of many things the family does together to help them function more effectively. We have not undermined the position of either the child or his parents. We have not taken sides but have preserved our objective role.

(10) *Giving children homework tasks is a way of both reinforcing the relationship the interviewer and the child are establishing and reinforcing the child's ability to observe himself in the interval between the first and the succeeding interviews.* Children of school age know what homework is. They also like to be thought about, by the interviewer, in the interim between the initial interview and the next one. I told Charlie I was giving myself some homework to do—some things to think about during the five days he was away from the office before our next appointment. "I'm going to think each day, Charlie, how you told me that when you get angry, you lose your patience and end up sometimes hitting Sissy. It was your idea to count to a million if she gets you mad, so you can stop yourself from hitting her. My homework will be to wonder how you're doing. You know, whether that million-thing works for you." Then I gave Charlie his homework assignment. "Your homework, Charlie, will be sort of like mine. Maybe you can keep track of how many times this million-thing works and let me know next time we talk. Okay?" Grinning, Charlie agreed. If the interviewer can help the child to observe himself more objectively, and therefore more accurately, he will have done much to help the child clarify his own functioning for himself. This is essential if the child is ever to learn more adaptive ways of approaching various tasks

and of relating successfully with other people. Such devices as the interviewer's "best guess" approach and the homework assignments are designed to strengthen this capacity for self-observation.

(11) *The interviewer should use play materials primarily to open up communication in a relatively nontalking child.* Obviously, there are a few children who are so fearful, so shy and inhibited, that the interviewer cannot meaningfully relate to them through feeling-oriented talk. I recall, for example, the very strange first-interview behavior of six-year-old Carrie Hammersmith. Her parents, both of whom were rather remote, cold, detached, compulsive persons, had earlier described Carrie's inability to relate with anyone, her muteness, and her panic if any of her playthings were moved ever so slightly out of place. From what they had said, I anticipated meeting an autistic child. In that first interview with me, Carrie accepted separation from her mother in a compliant, robotlike manner. She did not speak during the entire hour. Occasionally she hummed sounds that I learned only later (from her parents' description) were her accurate mimicking of the sounds made by the wings of insects fluttering against the windows of the family's home on summer evenings. Since Carrie did not relate with me at all that entire hour, the best I could do was, in effect, to drift with her as she wandered around the playroom. If she started a particular free-play theme—as when she carefully constructed a seven-story model of a skyscraper from a plastic building set—I would attempt to enter her play by handing her a few of the next pieces, commenting about her construction of the building as I did so. But even here, Carrie was not able to relate with me. Her play, and mine, did not open up our relationship, nor did it even open up communication. All of these behaviors were, of course, quite suggestive nonetheless. Carrie was, indeed, an autistic child.

For the children whose fears and inhibitions leave them in an emotional position more or less midway between the good talkers like Charlie and Beth and the mute ones like Carrie, free play often does serve to open up communication, at least in the initial interview. I start out attempting to talk directly with an inhibited child, but if those first few minutes are filled with more pained silences than otherwise, even as I inquire about nonstressful themes, I shift the child quickly off the stressful talking to drawing, to a game, or simply to giving him encouragement to explore the playroom on his own. "You know, Johnny, lots of boys and girls do different things when they first come here to see me—the strange worry-doctor. Some like to sit and talk about their worries and their fun times. Others like to wander around at first, sort of look the place over and see what they would like to do. I've got magic markers and paper to color on, there's that army set and some dart guns—oh, you'll see there's a bunch of stuff." An inhibited child often will begin to talk, usually about nonconflictual themes at first, as he settles into some kind of free play. I recall an anxious, inhibited eleven-year-old son of a local lawyer who presented himself as a relative nontalker. At my invitation, he explored the playroom rather tentatively, cruising about for perhaps ten minutes. Then, picking up a checker set, he turned and said to me: "How about a game of checkers?" We sat down and played, almost in silence, across the end of the work table. A fair player, Johnny won the first and the second games. I trounced him in the third. At this point he jumped up in angry tears. "Why did you do that? That's just like my dad! He always beats me! And that's not all—he says I never can do anything right!" We were off and running; communication was uncorked.

(12) *The interviewer finds some play materials more useful than others for the purpose of opening up communication.* Some evaluators have a combination interviewing room and playroom in which they meet with children of all ages, adolescents, and adults. In these combination offices, play items are usually kept in one section of the room. Others, like myself, have a suite of offices that permits a playroom (in which I have seen children from infancy through age eleven or twelve) separate from the paneled, carpeted, denlike inner office in which I meet with adolescents and adults. This separate playroom arrangement allows one to furnish and equip the room more suitably for younger children. The playroom should be set up to provide the child with a reasonable balance of freedom and protection. It should offer simple play materials appropriate to his age, items allowing both creative and aggressive expression.

The playroom I use has a tile floor. The furniture consists of a metal kitchen-sink cabinet (for water play and for storage of any special project, like a car model, the child may be working on during the treatment hours as we talk), two open-shelved metal cabinets holding toys and games, and the eight-foot-long oak kindergarten table with drawers and matching chairs mentioned earlier. This second-hand table has proved invaluable to me in working with younger children. I can sit quite comfortably at the child's level across the corner of the table from him as we talk, draw, or play games together. The table affords the child a great deal of working space, which often serves to promote creative expression of all kinds.

On one wall of the playroom is a four- by six-foot blackboard. This has proved very useful because it invites the child to chalk in all manner of sketches that, in a semiprojective way, reveal his conflicts, feelings, and defenses. Some inhibited children I have seen will often draw on the blackboard although they shun making a more permanent record in the form of a drawing on paper. Being able to erase their thoughts seems to encourage expression.

For the many children who do like to draw, however, I have three items that promote this activity. One is a large painting easel, on which glossy finger-paint paper can be easily clipped with clothespins. In the tray of the easel are a number of felt magic markers of different colors. These markers are often more effective than either crayons or tempera paints for the young child to use—they can be picked up, used, and dropped instantly. There is no delay in mixing, as with paints. The colors are bright and therefore appealing. And they glide onto the glossy paper, an effect inviting more drawing and encouraging more talking. The other items are two four- by four-foot bulletin boards, made from inexpensive wallboard, on two walls of the playroom. These hold dozens of drawings made by many of the children I have seen.

These drawings made by other children often serve as an invaluable aid to opening up further communication in the children I am currently interviewing. In an initial interview a child will frequently ask me who drew a certain picture on the bulletin board. This gives me an opportunity to tell him a story about the child who drew the picture. All children naturally wonder about the troubles other children may have that bring them in to meet with the interviewer. As we both call attention to these drawings, stories of all kinds of troubles these children have can open up. Occasionally a child will relate to a story told about another child in a revealing manner. "Well, gosh, that's pretty dumb—who would ever want to leave home, even for a little bit?" said one school-phobic boy of seven, responding to the story I told of a twelve-year-old boy, painter of a colorful tornado, who was always running away from home.

Other play materials I have found useful for furthering communication in children of preschool age are the easily manipulated play dough (all kinds of exciting shapes and stories can emerge from a can of that) and a variety of inexpensive animal puppets made from cloth. A younger child will frequently play out a feeling-packed drama with animal puppets, whereas he may avoid using the flexible rubber dolls and human-figure puppets also available to him. Apparently the humanness of these latter materials inhibits full expression of conflicts and feelings by many children. I recall one sturdy five-year-old boy angrily saying as he soundly spanked the bottom of the bear puppet: "Now, you listen to me! Not one more drink of water! You get to sleep, you hear?" One did not have to wonder where the boy had heard all that.

School-age children, both boys and girls, have a natural developmental bent toward learning, with all of its structure, form, routines, and rules. For them, I keep a variety of games (for example, Rattle-Battle, Booby-Trap, cards, pick-up sticks, Chinese checkers, regular checkers, Score-Four) on hand. Caution must be used, however, because too frequently the games take on a defensive function, permitting both the child and the interviewer to retreat to a relatively stagnant, non-revealing position. But occasionally, as indicated earlier, games are needed to open up communication in inhibited school-age children. Then a game serves as a catalyst for talk about other matters as it is being played. Or, as in the instance of the lawyer's son who blew up over a checker game, a game can serve another very useful diagnostic function. Only then did I learn —and in a way whereby this particular boy could be helped to see it fully, too—that he felt constantly threatened in an ongoing, relentless, competitive struggle with his father.

Taken together, these twelve ideas and techniques can facilitate the forward flow of the first interview with the young child. At its conclusion, the interviewer is left with early, but nevertheless definite, impressions about the child's functioning. He has talked with the parents, and he has seen the child once. Now is the best time for him to talk with the young child's teacher in order to familiarize himself with her impressions of the child and to compare his own impressions with hers.

The Evaluator and the Teacher. The interviewer should obtain permission from the parents to call the teacher. Most readily give it, but a few have definite reasons—some rational, some not—why they do not wish the evaluator to call the teacher at this point. This initial reluctance must be respected by the evaluator. Later on, since it is generally useful for him to collaborate with the teacher, the evaluator can reopen the matter, after he and the parents have established a better working relationship.

It is important, too, that the evaluator not call the teacher (unless, of course, the teacher was the one who initially referred the child) until he has been able to tell the child, near the end of their first interview, that he plans to make such a call and that he has the parents' permission to do so. The interviewer can make this announcement in positive terms that he has already helped the child to understand: "Charlie, you do remember my saying all of us—your dad, mother, you, me —were sort of working on your worry puzzle together. Well, there is someone else, I think, who can help us figure all this out, too. That's your teacher, Mrs. Snyder. I know you have certain feelings about her, and about your school work. And about the other kids in the school. So that's why I'll be calling her. She can help me understand some more about how you're doing in school. When I call her on the telephone we'll talk in private some evening—like tonight or tomorrow night—so the rest of the class won't know about it. And I'm sure that she won't tell other people that I called her to talk about you. No, this is private with you, your folks, me, and Mrs. Snyder. How does all this sound?"

Charlie could accept this, although he was somewhat rueful. He anticipated, I felt, a bad report from her on his work. In fact, the announcement by the evaluator that he intends to make such a call often opens up a child's true feelings about the whole school situation. For example, when asked about the rueful frown that my announcement brought forth, Charlie said: "Well, I hope you still like me after you talk with her, Dr. Looff. She gets pretty mad at me when I don't hand in my papers, or when I do mischief. In fact, I wonder if she likes me at all!" This gave me the opportunity to make the important distinction with Charlie that adults—his folks, Mrs. Snyder, and I—could love him always and like his behavior most of the time but dislike certain of his behaviors at other times. It was after this that we closed our first interview. As mentioned earlier in this chapter, Charlie left the office smiling. He and I both felt good about our beginning relationship.

Generally, I do not telephone a teacher at school for an up-to-date report about a child I am evaluating. Most teachers cannot easily leave a large class to pick up a telephone in a distant office and spend several minutes giving me the kind of data I need. Some clinics evaluating children mail written questionnaires to teachers, asking them to fill in behavior rating scales and to put down their own impressions of a given child. The problem I have found with a written form of this type is twofold. First, the busy teacher already has enough forms to fill out in her work, and she might therefore be inclined to give only minimal data on this additional questionnaire. And the questionnaire frequently does not allow much scope for the very important area of the teacher's feelings about the maladjusting child. It is of critical importance that the evaluator assess these feelings. They are important in a diagnostic sense, of course, because they frequently point up the underlying meaning and purpose in the child's behavior; they also play a significant role in determining how the teacher relates with the child, an important consideration with respect to his future in the classroom.

For these reasons—that is, to get their excellent data in detail and to ascertain their feelings—I call teachers at their homes. I find it better not to call a teacher before seven o'clock in the evening. Earlier, she is busy with family needs, possibly including the bedtime routines of younger children of her own. After seven she is more likely to be free to talk for fifteen or twenty minutes about a child. All the considerations mentioned in detail in Chapter 2 concerning what I do when a teacher calls me to refer a child also guide my behavior here as I call a teacher for the first time to obtain her report.

I telephoned Mrs. Snyder at her home at seven-thirty the evening of the day following my first interview with Charlie.

An older-sounding woman, Mrs. Snyder was obviously upset and angry over Charlie's negative, attention-getting maneuvers in her classroom, his chronic failure to complete many of his assignments, his sloppy work on what few lessons he did finish and hand in, his occasional attempts to take over the class from her control, and his aggressively assaulting one or another child on occasion. She viewed him in the initial part of our talk as "a severely disturbed, poorly socialized, aggressive child." It was plain, as Mrs. Snyder talked, that she was almost at the point where she felt she could no longer cope with Charlie's behavior. When I reflected how naturally upsetting such behavior would be to anyone, she added the comment that "in all my twenty-three years of public school teaching, he's been about the worst!" She went on to say that this was her first year back at teaching after seven years of complete retirement. "My husband's retired now. He's older, you see, and our children are grown. I wanted something to do, and we needed a supplemental income, so I came back. But Charlie has made me wonder if it's worth it!"

Her words and feelings over the telephone corroborated the impression Tom and Alice Russell had derived from meeting her directly—that she, a strict, somewhat authoritarian person, seemed to have a need to maintain absolute control over the children in her room at all times. I began to wonder during the call, how much the interacting factors of Mrs. Snyder's age, her own life-style, and the natural difficulty of taking up teaching again after so many years outside the classroom combined to exacerbate Charlie's problems in her room. Certainly these probable factors in Mrs. Snyder were not solely responsible for producing the boy's disruptive and underachieving behavior, since the Russells had indicated that they had somewhat the same problems at home with Charlie before he entered school. Again and again, Mrs. Snyder stated how much difficulty she had "gaining control over Charlie. He fights me for control, Dr. Looff. He's so stubborn in so many ways!"

Mrs. Snyder's anger and anxiety dissipated somewhat as we talked. At this point, she was able to give me excellent further data. She viewed Charlie's motor-muscular development and coordination as being advanced for his age. In addition, his drawings, in her judgment, showed evidence of good visual-motor skills. From this fact, she said, she had told the Russells at the time she summoned them for a school conference that she felt he might not be brain-damaged. Instead, she had told them that Charlie was a severely emotionally disturbed boy who needed prompt psychiatric evaluation and treatment. I asked Mrs. Snyder her estimate of Charlie's intelligence. She told me that the scattered quality of his work suggested to her that he was definitely underachieving, but that she had no idea of what the upper ceiling might be on his intellectual capacity. Her guess was that the boy had somewhat above-average intelligence.

At the end of our call, Mrs. Snyder told me that she felt she could cope most effectively with Charlie "by leaving him to work on his own the best he can. If I don't cross him, he's okay for most of the day." Because of the depth of Mrs. Snyder's still-present negative feelings about the boy and because of her needs and life-style and the boy's problems with which I was beginning to become familiar, I could only agree with her, at that point, that she had undoubtedly made the best management decision for the present time. I assured her I would be in touch with her again at the end of the evaluation to share my findings with her, to further discuss our views of Charlie, and to plan together for his management within the classroom.

Mrs. Snyder's report gave me an important new lead in understanding the misbehavior for which Charlie was being referred by her and by his parents. The boy, alone with me in our first interview, had been a bright, sensitive, well-related, altogether cooperative lad. None of the misbehaviors he was capable of exhibiting at school and at home were seen in my interview with him, even though he and I discussed these behaviors in some detail. Mrs. Snyder's report suggested why he behaved differently with me. Unlike his teacher and his parents, I had not assumed the posture of the authority figure, battling him for performance and control. The anguished report from Mrs. Snyder confirmed a number of impressions that were already taking shape in my mind from what Tom and Alice Russell, and Charlie himself, had told me thus far in the evaluation. These impressions were enlarged upon in my succeeding interviews with Charlie and his parents. They are summarized in their final form in the first part of Chapter 10, as my way of having to think through the final formulation of Charlie's case before I met with his parents in the follow-up conference that concluded the boy's evaluation.

In the next chapter, however, we digress from Charlie's case. There we meet the adolescent who comes in for his first interview with the evaluator.

Chapter 6.

Meeting the Adolescent: His First Interview

Establishing a Relationship. The initial interview with an adolescent is in many ways similar to that with the younger child; here too the evaluator must create an emotional setting within which the youngster can begin to feel free to relate and to share his needs and concerns.

The techniques that one can use to facilitate the forward flow of the interview with the teenage boy or girl are the subject of this chapter. They are not substantially different from the techniques used with younger children, with the exception, of course, of the use of play materials. (In this regard, I recall the scornful glance into my playroom by one thirteen-year-old predelinquent boy who, at my direction, was following me into my inner office for his first interview. His scathing comment underscored his dependent-independent, young child-growing man conflict: "Huh! Looks just like kid stuff in there!") Although the techniques themselves are similar for the two age groups, there are some crucially important differences in the ways they are applied by the interviewer. These differences result from the developmental differences between the two age groups.

The adolescent, regardless of the nature of his presenting problems, is always struggling, either successfully or unsuccessfully, with a range of developmental tasks—emancipating himself from his previous slavish conformity to his family's ways of thinking, feeling, and behaving; establishing a new, positive identity in his own right, a settled sense of self, a coming to know and feel what power he has in and of himself; turning outward from his family to establish himself as a participant member of a cohesive peer group; coming to grips with the physical changes and feelings that mark his pubescent growth spurt; discovering girls, or boys, and finding entirely new ways of relating with them; and mastering the demands of school, part-time jobs, extracurricular activities, hobbies, crafts, sports, and driving. All these tasks, with their attendant feelings, daily weigh upon the adolescent. They shape his moods, which are often mercurial, shifting in rapid, labile fashion. When he meets and masters one or more of these tasks well on a given day, the adolescent's joy and zest are keenly palpable. However, when he fails in a task, his feelings of disappointment, hurt, shame, anger, doubt, and even despair can be equally intense. Intense, too, at times is the adolescent's self-criticism, much of which is commonly projected onto others ("Nobody around here ever trusts me. They think I can't do anything right!").

The feelings attending any adolescent's attempts to meet and master these tasks are forces that simultaneously add to and detract from interviews with him. On the one hand, the intensity of his pleasure—or his anger and despair—makes such feelings readily apparent in any interview. Very little guess-work about feelings is called for. The interviewer need only sit, listen carefully, and observe. In the words of a physician's sixteen-year-old daughter I saw recently: "Gosh, nothing's a secret anymore! All my feelings tend to blop out on the table!" What an accurate description! Interviewers of adolescents do indeed tend to hear, see, and get caught up in "blops" of feelings—the adolescent's and, frequently, their own. In one way, this tendency for feelings to be intense and to show in any interview is a positive factor, since it frequently leads to rapid clarification of the meaning of a particular event to the adolescent himself.

On the other hand, this same intensity of feeling can at times be alarming, even very frightening, to an adolescent. At such times he often feels he has no more personal control over the eruption of feelings than he has over the eruption of acne. He feels vulnerable, at risk, very much on public display with his feelings. No wonder, then, the more insightful of our adolescents frequently say something like this comment from a sixteen-year-old boy: "Well, you know—coming here to talk about how I'm doing is maybe okay, in one way. But I feel so—you know, like the other day when I couldn't stop crying in here—like, well, ashamed. I felt like you could see right through me. I felt almost like I didn't have any clothes on, I was so embarrassed!"

Thus the adolescent's awareness of the intensity of his feelings and of his emotional lability frequently combines with his self-criticism to put him very much on the defensive—to make him feel vulnerable indeed to the scrutiny of an evaluator. In fact, nearly every adolescent, regardless of the nature of his problems, feels vulnerable in an interview designed to investigate his personal functioning. And nowhere is this feeling more apparent than in the initial interview. There the adolescent frequently behaves in a manner suggesting that he views the interviewer not as a friendly, collaborating professional but as a penetratingly discerning judge before whom he stands naked and defenseless. If we add to this feeling the fact that most adolescents do not ask for our services but are brought to us by troubled persons around them, we can understand the reluctance with which they come. This reluctance ranges from mild, bored antipathy through open wariness to angrily vocal rebellion. All these feelings produce behaviors that are apparent as the adolescent crosses the threshold of the waiting room for his first interview.

At the outset the interviewer should recognize these feelings and help the adolescent deal with them. Otherwise, they act like an ax handle in the wheels of progress; the interview cannot move forward. The adolescent will remain at least wary, if not openly hostile. Either way, he is relatively resistive, guarded, noncommittal. But if he can be helped to recognize and deal with his feelings about the referral process, the adolescent will have experienced early, tangible aid from the interviewer. This experience often enables him, within that initial interview, to move into areas beyond the referral process, into the realm of his own life events, relationships, feelings, and ways of coping with stress. The following story about Douglas, a fourteen-year-old tenth grader, clearly illustrates this.

In their joint interview preceding Douglas' appointment, his parents, Mr. and Mrs. Robert McTavish, vacillated between seeing him as a normal teenager going through a rebellious phase and worrying that he was a disturbed youth with significant internalized problems. Mrs. McTavish, in particular, favored the latter viewpoint. A plump, soft-spoken, middle-aged woman, she had grown up in a genteel household consisting of quiet, controlled parents, herself, and her two younger sisters. The emphasis in her home was on reading, music, education, and dutiful execution of work responsibilities around the house. Her own life-style shown as she related with her husband and with me in their interview, was that of a mature, concerned, somewhat inhibited woman. She was clearly puzzled and upset over Doug's behavior over the past four or five months. He was their first child, and only boy. The couple had two younger daughters, ages nine and six.

According to his mother's description of him as a younger child, Doug had been a consistent source of pride for her. He seemed to be growing up as a quiet, compliant boy who did his chores and was never oppositional and only rarely argumentative. Recently, however, his mood swings had disturbed her. Often, for example, after she had reminded him to take out the trash, he flared up: "Gosh, why does everyone have to pick on me!" In a black fury that alarmed her he would stamp out the back door, rattle the garbage cans with a vengeance, and slam the emptied trash container back down on the kitchen floor. Then he stomped off to his room, slamming the door. "Why," she said, "he's never closed the door on me before. I just don't understand it." Doug would stay up in his room, apparently reading, or playing "those awful hard-rock records," for several hours. When called from his room for supper, he would comply but would sit silently throughout the entire meal, his black brows ominously knit. "Why, he used to talk so cheerfully at the table," his mother said. "What's come over him?" Sometimes Doug failed to tell his mother that he needed to be driven home from an after-hours sporting event at his high school. As he walked later through their front door, he would angrily assail her for leaving him stranded. All of these changed behaviors and moods in their son clearly upset Mrs. McTavish.

Mr. McTavish, on the other hand, saw no real problem in Doug. "I know my wife is upset, Dr. Looff, but he's no different, really, than I was at that age. I had a close relationship with my dad. But I can remember sitting in our living room, studying my homework, and all the while boiling angrily inside toward the man. And, really, he hadn't done anything to make me angry with him. All he was doing was sitting there across the room from me, quietly reading his newspaper like he always did. And there I was, annoyed over the slightest rustle he made! Seems like I was looking for petty things he did, and blowing them up out of all proportion. I think I was just going through a rebellious phase, and, in my opinion, Doug is doing the same thing."

Mr. McTavish, a direct-speaking, more verbally aggressive person than his wife, showed many pleasurable feelings in their interview as he described how well Doug was doing in school (A and B grades in his subjects), how devoted the boy was to his favorite sport of wrestling (Doug was on the school wrestling team), and how well accepted he was in a close group of boys with whom he played neighborhood and church-league basketball. Mr. McTavish concluded his views concerning their son with the remark: "So you see, Dr. Looff, my wife really doesn't know if Doug is seriously disturbed or not. She thinks he has some kind of a communication problem. Our family doctor agreed with her that he may be disturbed. He recommended that we bring Doug here for an evaluation by you. Maybe you can sort it out for us."

At this point we discussed how they might prepare Doug for his coming interview with me by summarizing aloud to him all they had told me. In that way, I told them, Doug would have an honest, direct expression of their faith and pride in him as well as of their present doubts. They agreed to do this, and an appointment was then set for Doug for several days later. His parents indicated they would both accompany him to his initial interview with me.

On the appointed day, the three of them entered the waiting room in absolute silence. Mrs. McTavish looked strained as she pulled at a handkerchief in her hands. As she acknowledged my greeting, her words were hardly audible. Mr. McTavish was cordial but looked somewhat shaken, too. As we shook hands, he rolled his eyes slightly in Doug's direction, to signal me, I felt, that all was not well with the boy. Doug himself wore a thoroughly grim look. A swarthily handsome, dark-haired, dark-eyed boy of medium height and muscular build, he acknowledged my greeting with an almost imperceptible nod, shunning my handshake. His brows were knit together, his lips were set in a firm, straight line, and his jaw jutted forward slightly. The parents said, with what seemed relief, that they were going to a restaurant in the area for a late Saturday morning breakfast and would return for Doug at the end of the hour. They left abruptly. I indicated to Doug that we would be meeting in my inner office. Silently he followed me into the room and took one of the three interview chairs.

There he sat, stonily silent, his plaid jacket buttoned up, his stocking cap locked in front of him in a two-fisted grip. His facial expression remained unchanged. As I sat down in the swivel chair by the side of my desk, and started to load my pipe with tobacco, I said to Doug, "Well, I'm pleased to meet you and to have this opportunity to talk with you, Doug. But if you are in any way like I was when I was fourteen, or are like most fellows I know who are fourteen now, I'm not so sure you're pleased to meet me under these circumstances. Did your dad and mother discuss with you just who I am and why they wanted you to talk with me?" A brief, stony stare, then Doug blurted out an angry one-liner: "You're a damn head-shrinker!"

My response was a fairly long-winded one. "Well, okay, I can accept your word 'damn' because it's a four-letter one that says very honestly, I think, how you feel right now. There's an angry edge to your voice, and I suspect your anger was behind your silence just now and the jut of your jaw, too. That's okay—most fellows would probably feel the same way under the same circumstances. But your label 'head-shrinker' is one I can't accept, Doug, because it's not one I'd feel comfortable wearing around very long. It happens I rather like myself and what I do in here most of the day. Actually, the last head-shrinkers I knew were an Indian named Nah-Tay in Dick Tracy and some rather primitive savage types in the Smithsonian. I'm not really like that. I couldn't live with myself for long if I were.

"No, I'm a psychiatrist—and here, maybe, you can see how I have to explain myself to the little kids who come in here— you know, the very much younger kids who can't pronounce 'psychiatrist' yet [at this point I was demonstrating a younger child by holding my hand about three feet above the rug beside my chair], let alone know two beans about what I do and am interested in. For them I have to say I'm a worry-doctor, interested in the worries and problems all kids have growing up. For you bigger fellows, though, my task is easier. You've had a heap of growing behind you, and you already know very well what my job is. I don't have to cover the same ground with you. But let's get back to those feelings you walked in here with, and I dare say, still have stuck in your craw right now. Those feelings are anger, aren't they?"

"You're damn right," Doug replied, still angrily. "I didn't want to come here. Mom says I've got some kind of problem, but I'm not crazy!" My response, again, was a lengthy one. "Well, Doug, my heartiest congratulations to you—for what they're worth—on one thing. You at fourteen now have it all over me, back when I was this age. Like most fellows, I was pretty mad and upset when I was made to do something I didn't want to do. Only I couldn't always label the mad feeling out in the open, with words, and tie it into anything, the way you're doing now. In fact, I'm wondering if this is generally true of you most of the time—you can sort out your feelings accurately, label them, and tell others how you feel like you did with me just now."

Doug's facial expression relaxed somewhat as he shrugged a minimal reply. "Oh, I don't know. Well, maybe." Then a belligerent edge crept back into his voice. "Yeah, I think I know myself pretty well most of the time. Yeah, I do all right by myself." I agreed with him, quickly, on one point he had made. "Well, you're certainly doing all right by yourself on one very important point in here right now. You're absolutely correct, Doug, in saying you're not crazy. You know you're not psychotic, and I know that, too—from what your folks said about you when they were here the other day, and from the way you come across to me. No, you're not at all psychotic. But I know how it was with me at fourteen, and how it is with John and Mary right now. They're the two teenagers at our house. The three of us can have worries like anyone else, but none of us is psychotic, either. So here we sit. I'm the strange new psychiatrist you've never met before, sitting over here all bushy-tailed and eager to hear about what worries you might be having other than psychosis. And there you are, all mad because Mom hung a problem label on you and made you come today. This game could be a shutout. Or shall we scrub it on account of a threatening storm?"

Doug grinned faintly as he replied, "Well now! I'm mad at Mom right now, not you. You talk straight, more like my Dad.

Wish Mom would. She changes her mind a lot. I suppose she
fed you a line when she was in here. All about the big problem I am!" But at this point, heavy anger in Doug's voice had
gone. Annoyance was there, in a peevish sort of way. But,
clearly, much of his anger—reactive, or secondary to the referral process itself—had been drawn off by this time in our
interview. I felt the boy was now at a point in his feelings
where we could discuss, back and forth in a more objective
way, the concerns his mother had raised about him.

Accordingly, I asked Doug whether he was now feeling less
angry and perhaps, therefore, better able to join me in a discussion of how "all kinds of things are going for you." The
boy agreed he now felt more open, freer to talk in the interview. Furthermore, he felt, too, that most of his anger was
gone. "It's funny," he said, "it's like this at home. When I'm
really mad I don't say anything—just go off by myself." I
chuckled aloud, then said, "Well, Doug, you're right again.
For a few minutes there I thought you were so mad you
would really go off by yourself. You know, withdraw from
our discussion. Then I'd be left here without a partner, in
a no-good-for-anybody, one-sided talk." He grinned.

Since Doug was now ready to discuss his own functioning,
I felt it important to raise several crucial points which would
orient both of us to the remainder of this initial interview and
to subsequent interviews. "Doug, there are a couple of things
I feel are pretty important to guide both of us from this point
on—for the rest of this hour of discussion, and for whatever
number of talks we may have together in the future. Maybe
you won't mind if I take eight or ten minutes here to get them
off my chest. I hope these things will be sort of like a road
map we can use to guide our talking together.

"The first is that I usually find teenagers quite capable of
sizing up themselves—how they're doing, and their feelings. I
call this self-observation. It's like you're sitting where you are
now, and seeing Doug McTavish over in that other chair, taking a good long look at him, and describing him to me. Sure,
you may get hung up on a couple of points as you do this, but
that's my job as your partner in this talk, to help you over
the bumps. And some of this talk can get pretty bumpy—you
know, tough, or embarrassing, or whatever. But you won't be
alone if we hit such a spot. Many of us were fourteen, too,

once—and I'll feel free to throw in a yarn or two about how it was with me, or with John and Mary, to help you over the rough places, so we can really get clear how your situation is like mine was, or John's is now, or how it's different, as the case may be.

"Then, too, before we start rolling on here together, we ought to be clear about this whole business of confidentiality —you know, the business of privacy. There are some pretty open things like arguments going on in your home everyone knows about—your folks, you, and now me—that I ought to feel free to talk back and forth about between my talks with your dad and mother and those with you, Doug. These matters aren't secret. They're open to everyone's view, and so can be discussed openly, back and forth. This helps me, by the way, to help all of you get along better together sometimes. But there are often very private, very personal, secret thoughts and feelings you may talk over with me in here that you don't want your folks to know about. Then I keep them quiet, to ourselves. That kind of secret stuff stays secret. The same goes for your parents. They may have some secrets of their own I'm not free to share with you. And if I ever feel that what you tell me ought to be discussed openly with your folks— that it's not really secret—I'll tell you what I want to do, to get your permission to talk it over with them. That way, you know I'm no tattle-tale, and there are no surprises for anyone in our talks.

"The last thing, Doug, is something I feel pretty strongly about. It's hard to label this next thing without using a word that may not mean much to you right now, or it may. It's 'identity'—and by that I mean any teenager's coming to know himself in a settled sort of way, having a settled sense of self. This thing to me is 'the name of the game' of anyone's adolescent years. It's like coming to know what power you have in and of yourself, with real certainty. Teenagers build this power thing up from whatever they do. Or, sometimes, what they do doesn't give them much of a sense of power in and of themselves. Either way, it's pretty important. I think it's so important that it shapes up how I listen to you, Doug, from now on, and it shapes what questions I might ask to fill in your story of how you're doing. Now, before you get the idea I'm a windbag who can't shut up and listen, I'd better punt the ball downfield to you, and let you run it back awhile!"

Doug had listened attentively to this long orientation. In spite of its length, he, like many other adolescents with whom I've met, responded well to the concepts outlined in the talk and to the structure they provided, within flexible limits, for the flow of the interview itself. Doug picked up first on the "power in yourself thing," as he echoed it back. With real pride in himself gradually showing on his face, he began to describe—hesitantly at first, then, with verbal support from me, to the point of open role-playing—his beloved wrestling. "It's my thing, I guess," he said. He displayed rather keen insight into his own and his parents' feelings about his favorite sport. "Dad likes me to wrestle. He watches all the matches. Mom won't. She says she can't stand to see anyone hurt. I try to tell her it's safe, the way we're coached and all, but it's no use. She won't listen. It's like her feelings are made up already. You know—she's afraid I'll get hurt. Sometimes I get the idea she can't stand to see me grow up—like I should be a little boy all the time. But I like wrestling. I get a real good feeling inside from trying myself out in a match. Funny, it's still a good feeling even though I don't usually win! Maybe it's like your power thing. I mean, well—."

Doug looked somewhat embarrassed at this point. "Doug, go ahead. You're doing great. And you're on to something. Don't quit on us now!" "Okay," he said, a faint flush on his cheeks, "I really don't know what to call this feeling I get from wrestling. Maybe, well, once, when I was about seven, I guess, I was outside alone one night and I reached up and tried to touch the moon. Felt good then. That's the way it feels now—like I'm sort of reaching for something." A lump came into my throat, and I felt my eyes watering. "Doug, what you see in me are tears of joy. You've described in a fine way how it feels for you, or me, or anyone to stretch out, to really try yourself fully in something. No wonder you keep coming back to wrestling, even though you lose sometimes."

From there, we discussed in considerable depth his relationships with his parents and with his friends, his progress in school, and his ambition to be a physical education teacher of youths like himself. Doug felt quite definitely that his mother tended to baby him, to which he reacted with sullen withdrawal or openly angry outbursts. As I reflected his examples illustrating their mutual behavior back to him, it became clear that sometimes his mother did, indeed, overprotect him or baby him somewhat. But there were other times, I felt aloud to him, that he was feeling very self-critical, as any adolescent might and was projecting this personal feeling onto his mother, "so it comes out like she's on your back and bugging you." We talked briefly, then, of how he might watch his own and his mother's behavior more objectively, as he was beginning to do in the interview. "Learn to see it as it is, Doug. Sort it out. If it's really babying, you can diplomatically not respond to that, but reassure your mom it's your teenage thing and not to worry. And it may help to tell her the good feeling you get inside from wrestling, or whatever else you may do. But if it's your self-criticism, or your feeling anxious, or uptight, so that you've got thumbs-down feelings about yourself—then watch out for projection, accusing Mom of picking on you. That'll drive her up a wall, which doesn't help you any either because then she worries about this deep problem you've got or something. Really, Doug, from what your folks told me, from what you've said today, and from how well you come across to me, I'd say you're clearly not a disturbed fellow. You're a normal fellow through and through. But, as is the case with all of us who've been through adolescence, there could be some more understanding of you on your mother's part, and some smoothing out of your own reactions as you sort out what's really going on with you."

Doug and I closed that first interview on an amiable note, with the understanding that I would discuss his normality with his mother and father and that he and I would meet a time or two in the future to see how he was progressing in self-observation and in practicing some diplomacy in handling his natural feelings as he related with his parents and with others.

SPECIAL FACTORS AIDING THE FLOW OF
INTERVIEWS WITH ADOLESCENTS

It was suggested above that many of the techniques one can use to facilitate the forward flow of interviews with adolescents are in essence the same as those used with younger children. Specifically, these are: (1) reflecting feelings, (2) universalization-generalization, (3) pump-priming, (4) avoiding labeling feelings too early, (5) utilizing best-guess approaches, (6) assigning self-observational homework tasks, (7) feedback of impressions through the continuous use of summary, and (8) avoiding overidentification with the child.

These approaches and techniques can be as useful in interviews with adolescents as they are with younger children. However, there are some crucially important differences in the *ways these techniques are applied* by the interviewer in his talks with adolescents. These differences take their shape from the major developmental differences between the two age groups of children. Such considerations are at the heart of the following four techniques designed specifically for use in interviews with adolescents. Perhaps it is a misnomer to label them as specific techniques. At times, rather, they may represent special ways the interviewer applies the other techniques to his work with adolescents. All four of these factors were found useful in my meeting with Douglas, for example.

(1) *The interviewer talks with the adolescent on a more egalitarian level.* The younger child, regardless of his current problems, is at a stage of development in which he tends to relate to the interviewer as an authority figure from whom he generally expects understanding, warmth, guidance, support, and direction. Adolescents also need warmth and understanding from interviewers, but their emancipating status as teenagers leads them naturally to be wary of guidance and direction in an interview unless it is structured along more egalitarian lines. By this I mean that the evaluator conducts the interview more as a talk between equals. Comments such as "my job as your partner in this talk" are part of this approach. So, too, are the introductory statements the interviewer makes as he tells the adolescent that he views teenagers as generally being very capable of sizing up themselves, their life situations, and their feelings, and of talking about such matters. Such statements are generally very supportive for the adolescent because they respect the emancipation that is a developmental fact of any adolescent's life. In effect, by assuming this type of approach the interviewer shows that he respects the adolescent's more

independent position and views him as a capable historian, co-equal with himself in partnership in their interview.
(2) *The interviewer discusses carefully the confidentiality of his interviews with the adolescent.* In my introductory statements to Doug, for example, I felt that the matter of confidentiality had to be mentioned. In discussing confidentiality, the interviewer can make the important distinction between general matters—events openly known to parents, teachers, the adolescent himself, and the interviewer which can be freely discussed back and forth in various interviews— and specific matters, or secrets that the adolescent must be assured will be kept confidential between himself and the interviewer. Such a distinction was spelled out to Doug. Here again, as with the egalitarian approach, the early discussion of confidentiality respects the emancipating status of the adolescent. A younger child rarely questions confidentiality because he is in a more dependent position. In fact, to discuss confidentiality with him—although interviewers of younger children do respect this position, of course—generally puzzles him. "Why the big deal?" he may ask. But to the emancipating teenager, confidentiality can be a "big deal" indeed. I recall vividly, for example, the fury of one sixteen-year-old girl who denounced her mother's reading her diary while she was cleaning her room one day. "Who does she think she is—prying into my affairs!"

(3) *The interviewer's focusing on identity issues early in the initial interview can both structure, in an acceptable and egalitarian way, and facilitate the interview.* No one issue is more central to development in adolescence than personal identity. This was defined to Doug in my introductory statements as a settled sense of self, the teenager's coming to know what power he has in and of himself. By putting the identity issue this way, early in the initial interview, the interviewer focuses or structures the ensuing discussion along developmental lines the adolescent can understand, respect, and respond to frequently. I have found it to be a very useful approach in my clinical work with adolescents. Those like Doug, who do "have a thing going" for them, like his wrestling, understand immediately what the interviewer means and will talk of the activity, skill, or trait which brings such satisfaction and pride

in themselves. Those who do not have such skills, however, feel rather powerless in and of themselves. They, too, respond to the identity-defined statements of the interviewer, in one of two ways: they may show depressive feelings resulting from the partial loss of self which powerlessness implies; or they may show the often negativistic, sometimes semidelinquent overcompensatory postures assumed as defenses against their feelings of powerlessness. Therefore, an identity focus is a high-yield approach to use with adolescents. It is effective because it, too, is shaped by an important aspect of adolescent development.

(4) *The interviewer often can effectively support an adolescent by sharing himself in an interview.* Although an adolescent may derive support from hearing the interviewer say he once was a teenager himself, and presumably has lived through some of the same events, relationships, and feelings the adolescent is trying to describe in the interview, sometimes greater support is furnished by the interviewer's telling a personal story about himself at that age. If the story is offered in a fact-finding, let's-get-this-matter-quite-clear way, the adolescent is not offended, nor does he resent the story as an intrusion on his talking time. Instead, he generally responds with relief that his feelings are understood because he is now struggling with the same developmental issues. Or, if the interviewer's own story is off-base, his experience quite different from the adolescent's, the story may still lead to rapid clarification of the adolescent's own experience and attendant feelings.

For example, I recall the tremendous pain one adolescent boy of sixteen seemed to be experiencing as I asked him if we could talk a moment about the physical aspects of his development. Universalization-generalization comments I made, such as "you would have to be an extraordinary young fellow, Steve, not to have some worries over your body's growth and changes," had not supported him effectively. He was anxious, seemed somewhat sad, and talking was therefore exquisitely painful for him at this particular point in our interview. Then I told Steve a story of my own bout with very severe acne on my back over a four-year period of my adolescence, of my self-consciousness for many years over the resulting scarring, and of the empathic pain my younger brother and I feel currently as each of our teenage sons faces the same problem.

Steve listened intently and sympathetically. Then he openly teared, and, with a lump in his throat, he poured out his own tale. He felt that girls would never like him because of the scar left on his upper lip by surgical repair of a harelip earlier in his life. My tale had prompted his feeling-packed story more effectively than any other method or approach I might have used. I tend to use personal stories—my own, those of my adolescent children, or those of other adolescent patients— frequently, often in every interview. They are effective in facilitating interviews with adolescents because they are both egalitarian and empathic in approach. Most adolescents respect and respond well to personal approaches having these qualities.

Taken together, these four factors are useful *both in themselves and as ways by which the other interview techniques are applied.*

The explanation of these techniques concludes the discussion of the initial interviews with younger children and with adolescents. In the next chapter we turn to the evaluator's separate interviews with parents. These round out his understanding of the child's mother and father as separate individuals with their own life-styles, each an important model for their child's own development.

Chapter 7.

Separate Interviews with the Parents

In the six-interview comprehensive diagnostic study, separate interviews with each parent yield important background information about the family's history and about their feelings and emotions. Already somewhat familiar with the child's mother and father from their inquiry and from their initial, joint interview, the evaluator now has an opportunity, in the individual interviews, to explore other important areas of the family's functioning.

(1) *The evaluator comes to know the life-style—the basic personality structure—of the mother and the father.* In the separate interviews, each parent is helped to discuss important self-observational data covering his or her own functioning as an individual, including such areas as personal conflicts, characteristic ways of coping with stress (predominant defenses), hopes, aspirations, ambitions, and personal ego strengths. The interviewer also looks for further information about the value orientations and belief systems of each parent. He seeks to learn how each parent thinks, feels, and behaves as a result of social class, ethnic background, present religious affiliation, occupational status, educational background, social functioning within the wider community, and physical health.

This survey of each parent's personal functioning is developed in greater depth as the interviewer inquires about social background. Here, the parents are asked how they grew up—how they came to be the kind of people that, in their judgment, they are now. This leads to discussion of the relationships each parent had with parents, siblings, and peers, as well as an investigation of what important other forces shaped his or her life from childhood on. In this way, the social data required to produce a thorough diagnostic study of a particular child begin to take on a three-generation look. There is the functioning of the child himself, of course, and that of his parents. But there is a third vital element—the grandparents, after whom, in important ways that now affect their child's functioning, the parents patterned themselves socially to some extent. In effect, *the most accurate view of any child's social functioning is a three-generation one.* This broader personal and social outlook must be discussed by the interviewer and each parent together.

(2) *Each parent, alone with the interviewer, has important things to say about the marriage and the functioning of the other spouse.* In this regard, the interviewer investigates with the parents the quality of both the husband-wife and wife-husband relationships (whether reciprocal, dominating, parasitically dependent, and so forth), and the interaction of husband and wife as parents (degree of fit, reciprocity, cooperation, complementary nature of role behavior, and so forth). As he obtains information about these relationships and interactions, the interviewer begins to see the degree of cohesiveness or integration of the family unit. Specifically, significant subgroup operations within the family may come to light (for example, failure to respect the individuality of some, or all, family members by one person in particular; seductive behaviors; or scapegoating of the child within his family). The interviewer learns as well something about the equilibrium-disequilibrium balance within the family—what persons, events, and feelings tend to stabilize or disrupt total family functioning. And, finally, he learns the degree to which the family is integrated outward, into the wider community—how they fit in as a family, how others see them and feel about them.

(3) *Separate inquiry with each parent gives the interviewer further understanding of that parent's relationship with the child.* Thus both parent-child (for example, supportive, rivalrous, dominating, overprotective, seductive) and child-parent (for example, overdependent, hostile-dependent, symbiotic) relationships are discussed. In addition, each parent can provide further valuable data on the nature of the child's relationships with his brothers and sisters (rivalrous, dominating, dependent, parasitic, and so forth), and with his peers (same considerations).

(4) *The interviewer discusses the developmental history, the*

background of the child. In this area, valuable data on history and feelings are gathered by the use of the Developmental Questionnaire (see Appendix), the use of which was explained to the parents at the end of their initial, joint interview. They were urged at the time to work on this questionnaire together as a homework item between interviews. This approach gives them time to gather all the information, and in doing so they frequently clarify for themselves some important links between the past and the present functioning of their child. Thus the task is educational for the parents. It also saves everyone valuable interview time—time that can be better used to clarify any obscure points including feelings, about their child's growth that their answers may raise in the interviewer's mind as he quickly reviews the completed form with each parent. Generally, I ask the parents to fill out the questionnaire as soon as possible after their initial, joint interview, so that the completed form can be brought in by the parent first scheduled to meet with me after that time. The questionnaire is then available to me in working with each parent at the time of their separate appointments.

To show how these four areas of investigation are covered in practice, we turn to individual interviews with Charlie's parents, Tom and Alice Russell.

SEPARATE INTERVIEW WITH THE MOTHER

Alice Russell was outwardly calm and composed at the beginning of my individual interview with her. We met in my office at ten o'clock on the morning after my first interview with Charlie. Mrs. Russell's composure was in such striking contrast to her anxiety during the initial interview with her husband that I was moved to comment upon it. "Well," she said, "there's something about all of us, I guess, that I've learned so far from coming here. You see, Charlie's problems over the years had me so beat down, so upset, that I really couldn't recall a time when I wasn't nervous. I was always stirred up. It's not that he was hyperactive or difficult to manage all of the time—but when he was in one of his quiet moods, I stayed nervous waiting for the next bad spell. But, Dr. Looff, three things, I think, are beginning to happen as a result of our talks with you so far. I think they kind of go together to settle me down a lot."

Puzzled yet pleased over her new-found composure, I wondered aloud to Mrs. Russell how she managed to sort out such definite factors as her word "three" seemed to imply. In reply, she displayed again the capacity for insight and the orientation toward feelings that I had seen at the time of her original inquiry and later in the first interview with her husband. "When you asked us, the other day, to give details about Charlie's behavior, I realized as we were telling the story—or, maybe, after we got home—that there are just as many good times, like when he's really absorbed in reading or watching television, as there are bad. I had got in the position in my nervousness that I couldn't see the times when he was functioning better. And something else happened, I think. I had gotten doubtful, very much so, to the point I couldn't handle Charlie very well at all at the times when he lost control of his anger. I ended up, remember, up a wall, screaming or spanking, which didn't help either one of us a bit. Then I'd unload on Tom when he came home. I'd give him only the bad times Charlie and I had been in since he got out of school, and none of the good times. You see, I couldn't see the good—my feelings blocked me.

"For the past year, Tom almost hated to come home, in one way. All I did was paint a black picture and demand that he punish Charlie. And he didn't like doing that very much, I can tell you! So he left me with my miserable feelings. And I really began to resent his not supporting me with Charlie. But the other day, like I said, we had to sort out good times from bad for you, and I began to hear myself telling of some really very good times. No one had asked me to do that during this past year, when things have come to a head between Charlie and me. But you did. And I couldn't ask myself, feeling nervous and doubtful the way I did. Do you see?"

In response, I told Mrs. Russell it would be perfectly natural for her feelings of frustration, anger, and doubt to render her often incapable of providing needed external controls over Charlie's anger when his internal controls were lacking; that these same feelings would often lead to anticipatory anxiety about the boy's, and her own, functioning in the future; and that, as she had told me so well, the feelings blocked memory of the boy's capacity to function much of the time perfectly normally for his age. Essentially, I was summarizing, reflecting to Mrs. Russell what she had told me. She agreed that the summary was accurate. Furthermore, she seemed to gain renewed confidence, within the interview, from seeing that I viewed her as a capable, reliable historian. She then proceeded to outline the other two factors she had mentioned earlier.

"Since our talk together with Mrs. Snyder, Tom has been really made aware that Charlie has problems. Before that, he had only my lopsided word for it. And did I resent it when he didn't support me and implied I didn't know what I was talking about! But I can see his side of it now, too. He reminded me of that, on our way home from our first meeting with you. He told me he heard me talk about some good times with Charlie for the first time in over a year. He said it made him feel that I could see some better functioning in Charlie the way he often did, on weekends when he played ball with him. There's another thing I feel good about: ever since that talk with Mrs. Snyder Tom's tried to step in more and help me with Charlie when it looks like he's about to lose his temper again."

Just last night, she said, Charlie had become angry when the television set malfunctioned in the middle of a Jacques Cousteau program on the undersea world. She had become frightened, expecting Charlie to kick the set "in the face." But Tom had quietly got up from his chair and steered Charlie gently but firmly out of the room down the hall toward the den, saying as he led the boy, "I guess both of us hate to lose a favorite program. But until we can get the set fixed, let's see what the encyclopedia has to say about coral reefs." Not only had this help made Mrs. Russell feel good; it had led her to decide that perhaps she could handle Charlie in the same way—"and, you know, some of that old confidence I used to have years ago started coming back."

There was a third hopeful sign, too. This had to do with Charlie's response to his interview with me. "He told me he sure-enough likes you," Mrs. Russell said. "But what really pleased me was that he said, quite spontaneously, that you had given him some important homework to do—something about working on 'patience and papers' together. Charlie laughed and made sort of a second-grade joke out of it. He said, 'Dr. Looff and I are going to do pee and pee together!' And he did try to be patient, until after dinner and the television blew out, even when Elizabeth badgered him in his room and Snoopy upset his water dish and I asked Charlie to stop playing long enough to clean it up. Any other time he'd blow sky high! So, you see, I feel Charlie is starting to work on his problems himself. There's real hope in that for me."

By this point, Alice Russell had talked about several important shifts in their family's functioning. She felt supported by her husband's more active role in guiding their son, and she was pleased that the boy himself seemed to be somewhat aware of his problems. These shifts in the behavior of members of her family pointed up how, during the course of an evaluation, some people utilize the clarification of their mutual functioning and the emotional support afforded by the interviewer and themselves to work on their problems immediately. By doing this, families like the Russells reveal their relative stability, their cohesiveness, and their ability to adapt—to shift role behavior to meet and master interpersonal problems. Obviously, these families are not markedly conflicted ones; their adaptive strengths prove this point. At this stage in our interview, I reflected aloud to Alice Russell the conclusions I had reached about the family's capacity for adapting. I wondered, too, however, why she had mentioned earlier, in the initial joint interview, that Charlie had been a management problem for her from his birth. This question led her to begin telling me about her own upbringing, her courtship with Tom when both of them were in college, their marriage and struggles as a young couple, Charlie's birth, and the boy's subsequent development.

As she sketched in her personal background for me, Alice Russell looked relaxed, even pleased, in the interview. Theirs was a quiet, stable central Kentucky family, rather "stay-at-homish," as she described them. Albert Stevens, her father, a supervisor for thirty years in a local post office, was a warm, personable man well liked by his fellow workers and neighbors. More gregarious than his wife, whom Mrs. Russell described as a rather shy, retiring person, Mr. Stevens was "the one my younger brother and I looked to for fun. I guess I grew up sort of a mixture of both my parents. I didn't get the full measure of my Dad's sunniness, but I became less shy than my mother. You know, sort of in between them both in personality. Tom's a lot like my dad in his personality, except in their tempers. Dad stayed sunny, and Tom can really blow his stack sometimes when something doesn't work out the way he plans for it to. But I'm not knocking Tom altogether, you understand. In between his temper outbursts he is as outgoing, warm, and sunny as my dad ever was. That was what attracted me to Tom, you see, when we were both in college."

From these statements, and others she made, Alice Russell's self-concept emerged—her view of herself as a mildly shy, retiring person capable, however, of warmth in interpersonal relationships. She frankly said that she needed to lean on Tom as a more outgoing person to cover the mild degree of social anxiety she always felt in larger groups of people or with strangers. "Daddy carried the ball for us with others in our family, and I know I need Tom to carry it socially for me. But after Tom helps me get used to a crowd, I can settle down pretty well. Really, I guess I'm a lot like my mother, in that I need Tom to get me started in a lot of things. You know, I'm shy and sort of self-doubting, to a degree. On the other hand, Tom is a take-charge fellow usually."

This was why, Mrs. Russell said, she was so dismayed after Charlie was born. Puzzled, I asked her what she meant. Her subsequent comments about Tom, and herself, had remarkable relevance to the point of Charlie's having been a management problem for her from the time of his birth.

After a quiet courtship of nearly a year, Tom and Alice Russell were married the summer following their junior year in college. At the time, Tom was twenty-three and Alice twenty-one. Tom, who was from a farm family in northeastern Kentucky, had worked as a furniture salesman in a town in his area for two years after graduating from high school. During that period he saved some money, and he decided to go to college to study economics and business administration. These savings, plus their families' partial support, enabled the young couple to scrape by financially during their senior year.

From the very beginning of their marriage, they had similar views about children of their own. Even though they knew having a child immediately would limit their social functioning, both were, as a result of their own backgrounds, oriented strongly toward a family structure that was fairly small—parents and two children—and that functioned in an inner-directed, close-knit manner. This naturally led them to want a baby soon after they were married. They discussed the fact that, in having a child, Alice would not be able to teach as she had been trained to do. However, there was no conflict in this area, for Alice had grown up preferring to stay at home. Accordingly, she became pregnant several months after they were married. Charlie was born in Ashland, Kentucky, in August, three months after the Russells graduated from college together.

Almost at once, however, "the whole scene became one long-drawn-out nightmare for me," Mrs. Russell recalled. Actually, from her story I got the distinct impression that her nightmare began in the events of the three months prior to their son's birth. The couple had hoped Tom might secure his first sales position in Lexington, Kentucky, where salaries at the time were higher for salesmen than in most other regions of the state. Here they would have been near Alice's parents and brother and within one hundred miles of Tom's family. Here, too, the larger, two-university community offered them both cultural outlets and potential for Tom's later training toward his master's degree in his field. Unfortunately, however, such a post was not available for Tom in Lexington. After a frantic search for a job, he was able finally to secure a low-salaried position as a regional salesman with a farm machinery firm in Ashland, Kentucky, an industrial community on the Ohio River, fifteen miles from the farm on which Tom's parents still lived.

Alice Russell had only infrequently met Tom's parents and younger sister prior to their marriage. She liked his father, a quiet, stay-at-home man who cherished his garden and his beehives. However, her feelings toward Beulah Russell, Tom's mother, were quite conflicted. The older Mrs. Russell was a strongly domineering woman, often given to overreactive rages that somewhat frightened Alice during the few visits she and Tom had made to his parents' home from their college, which was two hundred and fifty miles away. In fact, Alice was rather pleased, during their senior year, that such a distance separated them from Tom's mother. Now, with their move to Ashland, as she described it to me in our interview, "I felt like we were moving under Mrs. Russell's gun barrel!"

"And that wasn't all, Dr. Looff," she went on, more and

more anxiously, to recall. "Everything bad seemed to happen to us all at once. The move up there in July, after Tom found his job, was bad enough. That summer was stinking hot, and smelly smoke from the oil refineries and the steel mills seemed to follow me around everywhere. There was just no relief from it. Apartments were scarce, and all we could get for what little money we had was this second-floor, tiny, dingy place. Hot, and no air conditioning! I sat and sweated out the rest of July and August until Charlie came—just a couple of weeks before Tom started his job."

At this point in our interview Alice Russell began to cry quietly. Her tears obviously indicated that, seven years ago, those events she had begun describing were indeed as troublesome as she said they were. Regaining her composure somewhat, Mrs. Russell continued her story. "Both Tom and I had hoped my mother could be with me for a few weeks right after the baby was born. But my dad had a mild stroke the end of that July and mother was afraid to leave him alone in Lexington. So she couldn't come up. And we just couldn't have Tom's mother in! There we were—no kinfolk, no friends, or anybody in a hot, strange town. Tom said he'd help me, but you know how that is, Dr. Looff. To make ends meet Tom got a second job the month we moved working six days a week as a brakeman in the Chesapeake and Ohio Railway switching yard there in Ashland. He worked the three to eleven shift. He did that for four years to stretch out his salesman's salary for us. So you see, he was on two full-time jobs. I hardly ever saw him. When he did come home he was exhausted—he just collapsed into bed. We couldn't go out, or anything. There I was—stuck home with the baby."

Alice Russell reached down into her handbag and drew out the completed developmental questionnaire. "You wanted us both to work on this, Dr. Looff. But you see from what I've just said Tom didn't really know anything much about Charlie for four years. Maybe that's a bit overdrawn, but it was more or less true of our situation then. I've had to fill it out myself. Charlie was a difficult baby to handle." In answering the questionnaire, Mrs. Russell indicated that she had had excellent prenatal care. Her pregnancy, other than the stressful events surrounding the young couple's move to Ashland, was without difficulty. Charlie was born easily, head first, in a local hospital after six hours of labor. There were no immediate problems with the delivery. Charlie cried lustily immediately and "pinked up" promptly. The baby, indeed, seemed to be off to a good start.

"But, Dr. Looff," Mrs. Russell said, "once we got Charlie home the rest of my nightmare began. It was so strange, in a way. There he was—an eight-pound lunker of a kid who, the pediatrician said, was the very picture of health. But there was nothing regular about him, in anything. The Dr. Spock baby book Tom bought me said that by the time a baby is several weeks old, he should be having regular cycles of sleeping and waking, digesting and eliminating, and, when awake, he should seem satisfied. But Charlie wasn't like that at all. Irregularity in everything was true for him all through that first year. It ran me ragged! And he was such a vigorous, squirmy, thrashing infant. You couldn't really hold him, he was so active. Why, I recall he banged around in his crib, on the floor, or in his playpen almost constantly when he was awake. Even changing his diaper was a trial—it's hard to powder a moving target! And Tom was no help. He was so proud of Charlie's being 'a grasshopper from birth' as he called him. But you can imagine how it all wore me down.

"And there was a real funny thing I began to see after about four months. The baby had this way of wanting to notice everything in sight—like he had to see, hear, and try to touch everything almost at once. I wondered then if that was what was making him so overactive. Sometimes certain things made him really overreact, like the color blue sometimes. One Sunday when he had a chance, Tom painted the nursery blue for me. Charlie really carried on in there after that, rolling and squealing in his crib. At first we thought he was reacting to the paint smell. But he kept on even after that wore off. Finally we decided it might be the color. When we painted his room over in an ivory color, Charlie seemed to settle down.

"By the time he was four or five months old I couldn't really predict any kind of a schedule for anything with him. Tom was away. His mother drove up from the farm just about every week to drop in for coffee. But all she did was criticize my handling of the baby. Between her and Tom—all he wanted was for me to keep that restless baby quiet so he could get some sleep—I gradually lost nearly all my confidence. And when Charlie got older, he kept on the same way. It got to the point, by the time he was a toddler, that I really didn't know if anything I was doing was right for him.

"But two things kept me going, Dr. Looff. The only two things that have kept any faith alive in me that I have any adequacy as a mother are the fact that Charlie seemed so outgoing, so friendly in spite of his hyperactivity and irregularity and this blue-thing, and having Elizabeth. What a joy she's been to handle! Elizabeth is a hundred and eighty degrees from Charlie. From birth she was a quiet, placid baby as regular as clockwork in everything. These two things have kept me going. I don't think I'm a total failure as a mother for Charlie, but for years I've just not known how to predict him. And I guess I need that to give me the confidence to handle him well."

Mrs. Russell concluded her interview by raising again the possibility that Charlie might have "minimal brain damage," though she reminded me that no pediatrician had ever felt that he had. But she couldn't "shake the notion, from what I've read, and from the way Charlie carried on all his life." As we closed the interview, I indicated to Mrs. Russell that part of my coming second interview with their son would be devoted to some screening tests for minimal brain dysfunction. Supported by this statement, and by my pleasure that she had been able to share with me so much additional information on background history and feelings, Alice Russell left her second interview composed again.

SEPARATE INTERVIEW WITH THE FATHER

Tom Russell related with me, in his individual interview at four o'clock the following afternoon, much like a friendly, bumbling Newfoundland pup. As his wife had stated, he had little information to contribute about Charlie's early developmental years. In an effort to put him at ease again, and to help him feel more adequate in his roles as husband and father, I steered our discussion to his sales career. Considerable time was spent in this area, tracing out his hopes and ambitions for himself and for his growing family.

Shortly after Elizabeth was born, an opening appeared for

a regional sales representative in one of the large farm-imple-
ment firms in Lexington. Tom's application for the job was
accepted. The family moved from Ashland to Lexington when
Charlie was nearly four. The move itself strongly supported
the couple. They were near Alice's parents and brother again.
Tom's job offered modest sales successes in his field. And he
had an opportunity to begin evening college courses that eventually enabled him to complete his master's degree in his area.
That degree brought him a sales consultant position within
his firm and regular annual increments in his salary. A year
prior to their coming to me for Charlie's evaluation, they had
saved enough money to make the down payment on a new,
large home in one of Lexington's newest middle-income sub-
urbs. All these advances, Mr. Russell indicated, "were settling
for all of us, to a considerable degree." However, even these
obvious strides ahead did not alleviate their difficulties with
Charlie.

At this juncture, I complimented Tom Russell on his ability,
just several evenings ago, to steer Charlie away from a temper
tantrum, and thereby strongly to assist Alice. Blushing with
pleasure, he indicated he was aware that he had done a good
job in handling the situation. Much of the remainder of our
interview focused on his growing awareness of Charlie's problems as we were all beginning to understand them now. Some
guilt showed too in Mr. Russell's feelings as he was able to say
at this point that he had for years not taken time to assist his
wife in the splendid way he did recently. "I guess I was pretty
selfish, those first four years. There we were, struggling to get
ahead. Me with two jobs, tired and cranky all of the time. It's
a wonder Alice didn't divorce me at the outset! She's really
a pretty good girl, Dr. Looff. None better in my book. But I
grew into a pattern of criticizing her handling of the boy instead of lending a helping hand. Maybe the scales are off my
eyes now, and you can help us both see if we're doing the best
for Charlie from now on."

On this growth-promoting note of Tom Russell's, we closed
our interview. Although I had gained most of the needed family
and developmental data about their son from Alice, and although Tom was not able to really say much about his own
life-style and personal-social background, this interview was
important nonetheless. It gave me the opportunity to assist

Tom to summarize his growing realization of the various ways he made an important contribution to his son's growing up. Acting on this note, Tom told me he thought he would be the one to bring Charlie to his second interview with me, scheduled for Friday, two days hence, at four o'clock.

Chapter 8.

The Second Interview with the Child

On that particular Friday afternoon, Charlie came into the waiting room just ahead of his father. No hesitancy slowed his steps as he came forward on his own to greet me; instead, a great grin spread across his face. "Hi! I'm back! Bet you missed me!" "Well," I replied, "I certainly did look forward to seeing you again, Charlie. It seems you're really pleased to be here. I'm glad of that. Maybe we'll have a chance to talk over that homework you said you might do this week." "Sure thing," the boy shot back at me over his shoulder as he marched on into the playroom. "Come on, Dr. Looff, I've got something to tell you!" "Well now," Tom Russell said, "I can see Charlie's settled in fine with you. Alice said he marched out of here in good shape earlier this week." Then, somewhat teasingly, he added: "Does your charm work best just with little children?" I laughed. "Actually, Tom, what you call charm works fine with kids like your son who are talkative, have clear insights into things, and know how to express their feelings. Lots of kids I see in here are not at all like that. But with children like Charlie, my job's easy. He seems bursting to tell me something. I'd better go on in and join him."

In the playroom, Charlie turned to me, smiled, and at once blurted out: "You know—that homework thing? I said I'd have to count to a million to stop from hitting Sissy, remember? And you said okay—so practice it and see if it works. Well, I tried it once, and it kinda worked and it kinda didn't. Well, the other night I was playing with my erector set in my room. Trying to build this gigantic [his word] crane that really works! Sissy came in, to watch me, I guess. But she got into the box of bolts and tipped them over. It made me so mad!" Charlie was becoming somewhat tense and flushed. "I screamed at her and I jumped up to hit her! But I remembered this million thing! So I counted 'one-hundred-thousand-two hundred-thousand-three-hundred-thousand-four-five-six-seven-eight-nine-hundred-thousand-one-million' and *then* I hit her!'' Charlie's expression at this point was a mixture of pride over partial utilization of a self-imposed control device and rather crestfallen awareness that in the end he had failed to control his temper once again. "Oh, well," I said, "win a few, lose a few. But I'm certainly glad you thought of it and tried to control your temper." Brightening, Charlie looked up from gazing down at his shirt buttons: "Maybe practice makes perfect!" We both laughed, and then we talked for a few minutes about safe ways of expressing feelings of justifiable anger, as we had begun to do in our first interview together.

By this time we both had settled into chairs across from one another at the end of the work table. Because Charlie was obviously feeling so comfortable with me, the time seemed right to introduce some special tests to him. These were introduced as "drawing and writing games, with pencil and paper, that help me understand some more things about you. You know, to let me see how you draw, do arithmetic problems, read, write, and copy designs." From one drawer of the work table I pulled out a manila "Diagnostic Folder" containing a copy of the Gray Oral Reading Paragraphs Test[1] and two sets of designs on 3 by 5 unlined filing cards that represent screening versions of both the Bender Motor Gestalt Test[2] and the Graham-Kendall Memory for Design Test.[3] From a second drawer I got out for Charlie several lead pencils and sheets of unlined, plain typing paper.

SPECIAL SCREENING TESTS

Because so many children referred for evaluation have chronic learning and behavior problems, the evaluator must always

1. William S. Gray, "Standardized Oral Reading Paragraphs," The Test Division, Bobbs-Merrill Co., 4300 West 62nd St., Indianapolis, 46206.

2. Loretta Bender, "Bender Visual-Motor Gestalt Test," the American Orthopsychiatric Association, New York, 1938.

3. Frances K. Graham and Barbara S. Kendall, "Graham-Kendall Memory for Designs Test," *Perceptual and Motor Skills, 11*, 1960, pp. 147-88. See also *Monograph Supplement 2-VII*, Southern Universities Press, 1960.

test for the presence or absence of certain specific learning disabilities that may or may not be contributing to the child's overall difficulties. If the child performs at his age level on screening tests involving reading, writing, arithmetic computation, and perceptual-visual-motor functioning, one can generally rule out problems like dyslexia (inability to read well because of a perceptual-visual-motor handicap), minimal brain dysfunction (a syndrome also involving perceptual-visual-motor difficulties across a wider range of the child's functioning than reading), and other chronic brain syndromes. However, if his performance is quite poor on these special tests (markedly below the average performance expected from children his age), the evaluator may suspect that the child has a specific learning disability. Acting on this awareness, the evaluator then plans to have the child tested formally by a clinical psychologist to determine the degree of his disabilities. The same considerations—screening tests, with referral for more definitive psychological testing if performance is poor— are applied by the evaluator to the question of mental retardation in the child.

It is just as important to go through the screening tests with adolescents, too. Generally I follow the same plan as with younger children, giving the tests during some portion of my second interview with the teenager.

(1) *Gray Standardized Oral Reading Paragraphs.* When this test is used to evaluate the child's sight-reading ability, the interviewer makes no attempt to formally score the child's responses. Instead, he notes whether or not the child reads aloud, below, at, or above grade level (the test paragraphs are numbered for each grade level, from the first through the twelfth grades), and whether or not the child makes errors typical of those made by dyslexic children as he reads. Dyslexic children generally struggle with all of the paragraphs, beginning with the very first one. In reading aloud to the interviewer (who sits beside the child to watch the printed sentences as the child reads aloud to him), such children typically make many errors involving elisions (syllables, words, or even phrases are dropped out), substitutions (another syllable, word, or even phrase is substituted in place of the one that was dropped out), reversals (certain letters, syllables, or words are reversed), and incorrect sequencing of letter sounds within words. The dyslexic

child's reading, accordingly, is extremely slow, choppy, and lacking in smoothness. In addition, he generally has a very poor grasp of phonics skills and cannot sound out words with which he is struggling aloud.

Charlie, on the other hand, found reading easy—to the seventh-grade level. He made no errors in reading aloud up to that level; he had a good grasp of phonics, showing an ability to more or less correctly sound out unfamiliar words beyond the eighth-grade level; and, through recall, he showed good comprehension of what he had read. Accordingly, I did not feel Charlie was a dyslexic child—in fact, he was an excellent reader.

(2) *Bender Visual-Motor Gestalt screening test.* This test is used by clinical psychologists as a measure of the child's perception and visual-motor coordination. Children with the particular type of chronic brain syndrome called minimal brain dysfunction (synonymous terms, in the past, have been minimal brain damage, minimal diffuse brain damage, minimal cerebral dysfunction, the hyperkinetic syndrome, or brain damage) appear to suffer from a variety of complex perceptual defects that affect their behavior and their learning ability in equally complex ways.[4] Considering the fantastic complexity of the brain, with its myriad interlocking circuits and groupings of circuits, it is not surprising for each child with this type of disorder to manifest a unique cluster of symptoms and to be handicapped in learning and in adaptive behavior (depending upon the nature of his environment and the magnitude of his defect).

Thus the perceptual-visual-motor deficits of children with minimal brain dysfunction show up in their poor writing, printing, and drawing. Their performance is poor and erratic when they attempt to copy geometric figures (Bender Visual-Motor Gestalt screening test; the Graham-Kendall Memory for Design screening test). Among the common errors they make on attempts to copy designs are distorted spatial arrangements, perseverations (attempts to compensate for poor drawing performance by task perseverance and/or innumerable and

4. Sam D. Clements, "The Child with Minimal Brain Dysfunction—A Profile," in *Children with Minimal Brain Injury* (Chicago: National Society for Crippled Children and Adults, 1964), 6-7.

meticulous tiny strokes of the pencil), "dog-ears," rotations of designs, and incomplete closures of lines on given designs. The third of these, the "dog-ears" effect, is produced on corners of designs, particularly; because of frequently associated synkineses, or motor overflow phenomena, these children cannot stop or start a line well. Thus they have difficulty in turning corners on a design or in changing directions of a line.

The child's total approach to the task and the time he takes, as well as the quality of the final reproductions he makes, must all be taken into account. The age of the child has to be considered, too, as one evaluates performance; for example, the central nervous system of the preschool child has not matured enough for him to copy the more advanced designs contained in both the Bender and the Graham-Kendall tests, which are used with school-age children and adolescents. Instead, the evaluator asks the preschool child to reproduce a circle (a child age three can reproduce a circle fairly well), a square (age four), a triangle (age five), and a diamond (age five or six). By the time a child is about eleven, however, he can generally reproduce rapidly and accurately all of the aforementioned screening designs put before him. For the child between six and eleven, therefore, the evaluator learns to gauge their average ability to reproduce such geometric designs through his experience with a number of children.

The designs I use in clinical evaluations are similar to, but not exactly like, the actual designs contained in the two copyrighted tests mentioned above (see Appendix). It is better to avoid giving a possibly handicapped child a "practice effect" through repeatedly exposing him to the same designs. If the evaluator uses the formal designs of both tests, he may inadvertently assist the child, through the practice effect, to mask his difficulties on the later, formal testing; therefore, when screening for the child's perceptual-visual-motor functioning the evaluator uses Bender-like and Graham-Kendall-like test designs. The ones I have found useful in my clinical work were prepared for me some years ago by Dr. Billy Ables, chief clinical psychologist of the Division of Child Psychiatry at the University of Kentucky College of Medicine.

In giving the Bender Visual-Motor Gestalt screening test, the evaluator sits beside the child. The designs are put before the child one by one and kept in his view for comparison while he attempts to copy each design on plain, unlined typing paper. The paper must be unlined; lined paper might assist the perceptual-visual-motor handicapped child line up his drawings, an effect that might therefore mask his real difficulty. When I gave this screening test to Charlie Russell, he copied all the designs rapidly and accurately. Occasionally, a child will make small errors in reproducing one or more designs. If this occurs, he is asked to compare his design with the stimulus design. If the child can perceive his errors, tell the differences, and correct them, one may conclude that his perceptual-visual-motor functioning is intact.

(3) *Graham-Kendall Memory for Design screening test.* As indicated above, this particular test, like the Bender test, gives the evaluator another measure of the child's perceptual-visual-motor functioning. The Graham-Kendall screening designs I use (see Appendix) are drawn up in a set, on plain, unlined 3 by 5 filing cards. In administering the test, the evaluator again sits beside the child. The child is told to "look at this design until you know it in your head. Take all the time you want. When you know it, tell me, and I'll hide the card so you can't see it. Then you copy the design as you remember it on your paper" (plain, unlined typing paper). After the child has completed drawing each design, he is again shown the stimulus design and asked to compare it with his drawing. If he has made errors, he is asked to tell about these and to correct them if he can.

Some children with minimal brain dysfunction (with its attendant perceptual-visual-motor deficits) can accurately perceive their errors on copying the Bender and the Graham-Kendall screening designs but, because of their poor motor performance, cannot correct their perceived mistakes. For example, one very bright eleven-year-old boy with significant perceptual-visual-motor deficits told me in tears, as he unsuccessfully struggled to correct his rendering of one of the Graham-Kendall designs for the third time: "Dr. Looff, I can see what I'm supposed to do here. You've got a square here, with a parabola curving down from the upper left-hand corner to the lower right-hand corner. But I can't make my hands do what my eyes see!"

Other children with minimal brain dysfunction may be

unable to perceive the distortions between the standard design stimuli and their reproductions. In such instances, we cannot say from these design tests alone whether or not they have motor damage, because with the visual function impaired they cannot get the design gestalt into the motor system without distortion. Thus these particular children may have visual and motor, or only visual, damage. Differentiation depends on further neurological examination, including visual testing, and on the data derived from a variety of psychological tests which tap visual-motor functioning. Unlike these children, Charlie had no difficulty copying the Graham-Kendall screening designs from memory. And, as on the Bender test, he was able to perceive and accurately correct what few errors he made.

(4) *Draw-a-Person test and Kinetic Family Drawings.* Some children, when asked to do so at the end of their first interview, will bring in to the next interview drawings of people they have made at home or in school. Others, who have not done so, can be asked to "draw a person" during the interview. Human-figure drawings often give the evaluator data in four important areas of a child's functioning: (1) the child's psychosexual identification may be perceived—generally, but not invariably, the child will draw a child or adult of his own sex when he is asked simply to "draw a person"; (2) the amount of detail the child puts on a human-figure drawing is a rough measure of the performance aspect of his intellectual functioning—the brighter the child, the more detail, generally, he puts into his drawing;[5] (3) the form quality of his drawing is another check on his perceptual-visual-motor functioning; and (4) the child's free associations (made at the interviewer's request) to the human figure he has drawn may reveal his worries, fears, and ways of coping with stress, as well as conflict-free spheres of his functioning.

Some children, when asked to draw a person, will draw not one but several persons interacting together in some form of story. Charlie's "watered-down picture," as he titled the drawing he had made at home and brought with him to his first interview, is an example. Such drawings illustrate the same

5. Florence L. Goodenough, "The Measurement of Mental Growth in Childhood," in *Manual of Child Psychology*, ed. Leonard Carmichael (New York: Wiley, 1946), Ch. 9, pp. 450-75.

four areas of the child's functioning mentioned above. Another example is the sketch made in her second interview by six-year-old Karen, a pale, willowy, chronically anxious child who was referred by her teacher and parents when she developed an acute school-phobic reaction at the beginning of the first grade. Like most other school-phobic children, Karen was markedly troubled with separation anxiety, the emotional hub around which her symptoms of headache, nausea, vomiting, and school refusal turned. In her drawing she depicted these concerns, as well as her beginning awareness that the separation anxiety involved her mother as well as herself. Her drawing was of "fall leaves who have sad faces because they are falling away and leaving the mother tree. And the mother tree is just as sad because her children are leaving her."

Obviously, the rich associations made by children like Charlie and Karen with their drawings are an invaluable additional source of semiprojective data concerning underlying conflicts. Children often make these associations spontaneously, as did Charlie and Karen. Others, less spontaneous, can be asked after they complete a human figure drawing: "Let's see, that's a pretty good picture. And I guess there must be a pretty good story that goes with it—you know, kind of a pretend, make-up story to go with your picture. Would you say you've made a boy or a girl, a man or a woman?" (Nine-year-old Billy, a dyslexic child, picked "a boy" in response to my asking him about his completed drawing.) "Okay, so this is a boy. How old would you say he is?" ("Thirteen," Billy replied.) "I guess he should have some sort of name. What do you think you'd like to call him?" ("Jimmy.") "Well, I guess Jimmy likes to do certain things, like all boys do sometimes. I wonder what he likes to do especially?" ("Well, he likes sports, especially basketball, and he likes to go fishing with his grandfather down on their farm.") "Okay, well I suppose like all boys he has some unhappy times, too—you know, tough times. I wonder what might worry this Jimmy?" ("He doesn't like to be teased at school, when the kids call him 'four-eyes' because he wears glasses, and when they giggle because he can't read well out loud, in front of everybody. That makes him sad inside all day long.") Previous to these feeling-oriented, revealing associations, Billy had said very little about his own reading difficulties, even

when he had floundered in attempting to read aloud the Gray
Oral Reading Paragraphs.

Some children may reveal troubled feelings stemming from
conflict situations if they are asked to produce a Kinetic
Family Drawing.[6] The evaluator may ask the child to make
such a drawing in the interview or to produce one at home
and bring it to a later session. The instructions to the child
are simply to "draw all the members of your family doing
something together." Even conflicted children will often
choose to draw a conflict-free family situation. Others, like
seven-year-old Angela, may reveal significant disturbances in
family relationships and their own functioning. Angela had
been referred through her second-grade teacher, who was
concerned that this bright girl did not do her assigned work
but instead sat around all day in class masturbating while
engaged in staring-out-the-window fantasy. In one of her later
interviews Angela, who related with me in a coquettish, dramatic way, said she daydreamed about a handsome Prince
Charming who would one day ride in on a large horse and
take her away as his captive bride. Angela's mother was a
quiet, mildly depressed woman who was often too tired and
emotionally exhausted to relate well with her bright, eager
daughter. On the other hand, Angela's father was a large, enthusiastic, handsome man who rationalized his and his daughter's seductive ways of relating with each other by saying, in
his individual interview with me, "I have to be available to
her since my wife can't be." When asked to produce a kinetic
family drawing, Angela brought in a picture she had made of
a seven-story building on fire. Her mother, she said, might be
overcome with smoke and never get out in time from the
kitchen on the first floor. Angela herself was leaning out a
seventh-story window calling loudly for help. And her father,
a fireman in the drawing, was rushing toward the house with
a long ladder to effect Angela's rescue. Thus her drawing
paralleled and further highlighted the unresolved oedipal
psychodynamics operating in all three family members that
were also being pointed up by the other interview data.
Kinetic family drawings, as their name implies, often usefully

6. R. C. Burns and S. H. Kaufman, *Actions, Styles and Symbols in Kinetic
Family Drawings: An Interpretive Manual* (New York: Brunner/Mazel, 1972).

depict the child's conflicted or nonconflicted ways of relating within the family itself.

(5) *Examples of writing and arithmetic computation.* From the recent school report obtained from the child's teacher, the evaluator usually knows how well the child is progressing in reading, spelling, handwriting, verbal comprehension, vocabulary development, and arithmetic computational skills. Generally, the children said to be good readers by their teachers, and found to be so through their interview performance on the Gray Oral Reading Test, are good spellers as well. To check this, the evaluator dictates a few grade-appropriate words and sentences for the child to write down. Children with dyslexia and/or a perceptual-visual-motor deficit central to the problems of minimal brain dysfunction do poorly on spelling. They frequently reverse letters, syllables, and whole words on paper when they are asked to write down such visually paired letters as "small b and d," "small m and n," and "small p and q," or the words "saw and was," "not and to," and "bad and dad," to cite just a few examples. The special sentence I use for dictation has in it a range of spelling words for all ages of children, and it is constructed in such a way as to magnify the types of errors made commonly by dyslexic children. It is: "The boy has a new blue ice machine." Nine-year-old Billy, the dyslexic child cited above, wrote this dictated sentence down in the following manner:

dog hob a near blew si megshen

On the Gray Oral Reading Test, Billy had great difficulty reading even the first- and the second-grade paragraphs. His performance was choppy and hesitant, with frequent reversals, elisions, and substitutions of letters and syllables. Aware of his own reading difficulty, Billy was quite stressed, in his second interview, by this school-type task of writing a sentence or two. Tears came to his eyes, and when this evidence of his inward pain was reflected to him, he confirmed the conclusion that he had great difficulty reading. Furthermore, he compared himself unfavorably with the other children in his class, who were much better readers. In this way Billy was very sensitive to his own learning problem.

In addition to having the child spell words and sentences, the evaluator asks him to work a few grade-appropriate arithmetic problems, in order to check on his computational skills. Generally, I first ask the child what kind of math problems he has been doing in school; then I ask him to write down a few examples for me and to work them. In this way I avoid giving the child problems that may be beyond his skills and level of training. The reason for checking computational skills is that some children with perceptual difficulties may exhibit them in the form of a dyscalculia, or inability to do calculations well with number symbols.

(6) *Time-spatial orientation tests.* Many children with perceptual-visual-motor deficits do poorly compared with their peers on questions related to their perception of themselves in relation to time and space. Most younger children of normal ability have no trouble with casually introduced questions such as, "Let's see, how did you get here today, Charlie?" ("Mom picked me up at school in our car and we drove right here.") "Okay, what's your best guess, Charlie, how far it is from your school down here to the office?" ("I dunno—maybe a mile." His answer was approximately correct.) "How long would you say it took you to drive down here?" ("Oh, about fifteen minutes. We would have come sooner, but Mom had trouble with the car in the parking lot at school. Guess she flooded it or something. And then we hit a lot of traffic at the shopping-center light.") "Gee, you're pretty good at judging time, Charlie. Now let's see how you do on judging weight and distance. About how tall are you now?" ("Oh, I dunno—maybe fifty-two.") "Fifty-two what?" ("Inches, I mean.") "I see, and about how much do you weigh now?" ("That's easy. We have a scale in the bathroom and I weigh in there every morning. It's sixty-one pounds now!") "Well, what would be your guess how much I weigh, and how tall I am?" (As I stood up from my chair, Charlie looked me over and replied: "Oh, you're shorter than my Dad who is over six feet tall, so I guess maybe you're five-and-a-half feet tall. And I guess you weigh maybe over a hundred pounds.") Charlie's

answers were reasonably close to my height of five feet nine inches and my weight of 145 pounds.

On the other hand, a child with perceptual-visual-motor deficits may have great difficulty with time-spatial orientation questions. Billy, the dyslexic boy mentioned earlier, also had some perceptual-visual-motor problems that made it difficult to answer the same questions I had put to Charlie. Billy's best guess was that it took "two minutes" to go "one yard" from his home on the bus (the actual four miles to his school). He was not certain how many feet were in a yard. Although he hadn't measured his height, Billy guessed he "maybe was two tall." When pressed for the omitted unit of measurement (such omissions are fairly common errors made by children with perceptual-visual-motor deficits), Billy answered "two inches tall." He guessed my height at "four yards."

(7) *Screening tests for mental retardation.* Various verbal and performance aspects of a clinical interview with a child permit the evaluator to make an estimate of the child's intellectual functioning. There are three aspects of a child's overall verbal performance—itself reflective of the child's intellectual capacity—that should be considered from his spontaneous talk in the interviews: his vocabulary level; his general fund of information; and the abstract way in which he uses language. A bright child generally knows a great deal about many things and expresses this knowledge through well-chosen words in abstract ways. His vocabulary is rich and his language usage colorful. This was certainly true of Charlie, for example. On the other hand, the child functioning at a retarded level generally uses only a few simple words; his speech is rather colorless and monotonous, and his verbal expression is concrete rather than abstract. Such impressions about the verbal performance of a particular child are frequently corroborated, as mentioned earlier, by his performance in drawing (richness or sparseness of detail).

Some intellectually retarded children, however, may have become rather facile in their use of spoken language. The input of language usage by others around them has enabled them to memorize certain words and phrases which they use with peers, parents, teachers, and interviewers in socially adaptable ways. If these seemingly intellectually average children were judged solely on the basis of their vocabulary level, their intellectual deficits might not spontaneously come to light. Only by asking such children to define some of the larger words they are using, and comparable other words, by listening carefully for the abstract or concrete quality of their language usage, and by checking on performance aspects of intellectual functioning as measured approximately from the amount of detail put in drawings can the evaluator tell whether such children may be intellectually retarded.

The case of eleven-year-old Timothy, son of a banker, is instructive. He was referred to me several years ago because of chronic learning and behavior problems. Both his parents and his teachers through the years felt that the boy was an underachiever. His vocabulary development and language usage suggested to them that he was clearly of above average intelligence and therefore able to do the work demanded of him in school, if he would just buckle down and try. His parents had thoroughly tutored him each evening for years. Little was accomplished in these frequently tear-soaked, angry sessions. Clearly, Tim's parents saw the boy as an oppositional child who just wouldn't learn.

Therefore, a crucial question about Tim's functioning, in terms of school adjustment and of his parents' expectations of him, was his level of intelligence. But this was difficult to judge in talking with him. His middle-class values and appropriate behavior, coupled with occasionally good vocabulary use, led me at first to overestimate his ability. But when he was asked for certain specific information, as in definitions, his language performance was clearly below that of his peers. For example, he gave the names of the months when asked the four seasons of the year; he did not know the number of stars in the United States flag, nor what they stood for; and he responded that the stomach's function was to give you air. For an eleven-year-old boy, these verbal responses were highly inferior ones. Corroborating these verbal deficiencies were the sparseness of detail and the generally poor form quality of Tim's human-figure drawing:

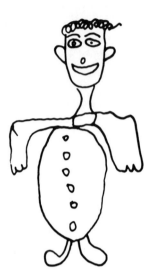

Later, when Tim was tested by a clinical psychologist, his intellectually retarded functioning was further defined. His performance on the WISC (Wechsler Intelligence Scale for Children, an instrument used frequently by clinical psychologists to measure a child's intellectual functioning) indicated a retarded to borderline level of functioning (total IQ of 68-70 on the WISC; verbal IQ score 67-70; performance IQ score of 75).

REVIEW OF THE CHILD'S MENTAL STATUS

In school-age children, borderline psychotic or true schizophreniform psychotic disorders[7] may occasionally be encountered. The onset of these disorders may be gradual, with

7. Schizophreniform disorders in school-age children are discussed in the *Group for the Advancement of Psychiatry Report No. 62*, pp. 254-56.

neurotic symptoms appearing first, followed by marked and primitive denial and projection, looseness of associations in thought processes, concretistic thinking, low frustration tolerance, hypochondriacal tendencies, and intense temper outbursts. Later developments in these disorders may include marked social withdrawal, intense involvement in fantasy, autistic behavior, emotional aloofness, true disorders in thinking, and a breakdown in reality testing.

In these children, regression is ordinarily not as marked as in schizophrenic adolescents or adults. True hallucinations are not commonly recognized as such until the later school-age period or adolescence. This may be due in part to the fact that, in the early school-age child, we normally expect to see fantasy and some persistence of magical thinking, making it difficult to be certain about such phenomena. Bizarre behavior and stereotyped motor patterns, such as twirling, are frequently present. Some of these children show sudden and wild outbursts of either aggressive or self-mutilating behavior, exhibit inappropriate mood swings, and make suicidal threats and attempts. Ideas of reference, dissociative phenomena, somatic delusions, catatonic behavior, paranoid thinking, and other manifestations like those seen in psychotic adults and adolescents may occur.

Ordinarily, conclusions about disturbances in the school-age child's thinking (apropos of looseness of associations in his thought processes and primitive denial and projection involved in ideas of reference, paranoid thinking, and even true delusions and hallucinations) are drawn by the evaluator from the child's spontaneous speech during the interviews. No special testing is usually required to uncover disturbances of thought in the truly psychotic child or adolescent. However, the evaluator must be alert to the possibility that a borderline or marginally psychotic child may not show the extent of his frightening fantasies, and the corresponding disturbance in his thinking and associated reality testing, in a rather structured face-to-face interview designed to investigate several areas of his functioning. It is only when the borderline psychotic child is asked less structured questions—about his associations to a picture he has drawn, for example—that the depth of his fantasies may be tapped and the looseness in his thinking revealed. This was demonstrated in my testing of Peter Schlatz, an eleven-year-old fifth-grade boy who was referred to me some time ago by his parents on the insistence of school authorities. Although his teachers felt he probably had superior intelligence (confirmed later on the WISC), Peter was failing in his work because of increasing social withdrawal into a private world of reverie from which he could not be dislodged to complete his school assignments. In his first interview with me, the boy related in an anxious, overly dependent manner. An intelligent, emotionally sensitive lad, he talked clearly of wanting to please his mother by being her constant companion and by responding to her constant, controlling directions in dutiful, compliant, submissive ways. He spoke of her as a protector for him against the angry, harshly critical ways of his father (in actuality a cold, aloof, compulsive person), who continually placed great pressure upon Peter to excel at intellectual pursuits. In other face-to-face, structured interviews Peter spoke clearly about his varied interests. His perceptiveness and the wide range of topics about which he had something intelligent to say made him a fascinating and pleasant child with whom to work. His whole mode of interaction, however, had a rather anxious, forced quality to it, as if he were whistling in the dark and simply had to keep talking to ward off his fears.

These fears emerged in some depth, revealing some beginning looseness of association in thinking and partial loss of reality testing, as Peter more and more anxiously associated freely to some human-figure drawings he made for me at the beginning of our second interview. One figure, half man and half bird, he designated a "scople bird—a female bird that comes down and sucks your blood out!" The name he attached to this creature was his own neologism. With mounting anxiety, he went on to say that the "scople bird" was a member of a Communist gang bent on destroying the individuality of people on earth, boys particularly. The bird had allies, Peter said, in the form of other, even more terrifying predatory creatures waiting to complete this destruction if the "scople bird" failed in its primary mission. Peter also made up a name for a male fish, a "copal," which "eats fish smaller than itself, but only when it's hungry. It's got crablike pinchers, and comes up close to you and bites and really hangs on. He gets your blood out because he lives on blood." The percepts themselves, even when taken as general concepts for "bird" and "fish," seemed to me of poor form quality and appeared unrelated, except in Peter's private fantasy, to anything actually present. Percepts as disturbed and affectively laden as this often indicate a thought disorder, either incipient or current, in a school-age child.

Peter was also intrigued by great historical figures. This interest was put in quasi-scholarly terms and hence was rewarded by his father, but it also illustrated the extreme anxiety the boy experienced in interacting with people. It seemed that by reading and daydreaming about historical figures, Peter was able to experience fantasy contact with people; yet they remained inanimate and at a distance from him and therefore were safe. He seemed reluctant to face social interaction even when it was placed in a historical setting. For example, he drew two human figures who belonged to the German nobility. Although he proceeded to describe their physical appearances in great detail, Peter was never able to make up stories telling how these people thought and felt. When I asked him to tell me a story about how these people interacted with one another, Peter simply was unable to do so, even when pressured. He could only add more historical detail about one or the other. Although these details sounded almost believable, those which had any basis in fact were confused and distorted, and most had no such basis. This example pointed up to me the distortion of reality that Peter had developed in his attempts to meet his parents' demands.

Peter was experiencing great anxiety and confusion, then, concerning both the real world and his own fantasy life. He appeared to be developing some very frightening, distorted fantasies, but he still attempted to justify them by referring them to supposedly real things. He tried to order his world and to shut out some of the disturbing affect by losing himself in stories about historical figures. In this way he could make vicarious social contact without the fear aroused by normal social interaction. It was apparent that Peter was retreating from social contact into a fantasy world which had less and less correspondence with reality. Diagnostically, I thought of him as having a borderline schizophreniform psychotic disorder.[8]

8. *Ibid.*

In addition to considering the possible presence of a thought disorder in a school-age child or adolescent, the evaluator is alert to possible disturbances in the sensorium of children he is asked to see in a hospital setting. Children with acute brain disorders associated with intracranial infection, systemic infection, drug or poison intoxication, alcohol intoxication, trauma, circulatory disturbance, certain types of convulsive disorder, metabolic disturbances, and certain disorders of unknown etiology (such as multiple sclerosis) commonly exhibit some degree of clouding of consciousness. In general, these acute brain disorders in children, as in adults, produce a delirium involving a disturbance in awareness as the result of the alteration of cerebral metabolism. The symptoms may be gross and easily identifiable, characterized by mildly agitated and confused behavior and hallucinatory experiences, the latter arising from misperception of stimuli in the environment. They may also be subclinical, however, with subtle disturbance in awareness or mildly stuporous states, withdrawn behavior, or irrational fears.

Finally, the commonly present deficits in recent memory as opposed to remote memory function of a child with a chronic brain syndrome may be tested through the use of forward and reverse digit-span or by the child's recall after a five-minute interlude of a story told him by the evaluator.

In Charlie Russell's meeting with me that second hour, his stories and fantasies were tightly organized, revealing no looseness of associations or lapses in reality testing. His sensorium was not clouded: he was firmly in interpersonal context in time, place, and situation. In addition, his memory functioning, both recent and remote, was accurate; this was revealed spontaneously in the many events and dates he discussed as we talked together.

FANTASY MATERIAL

For preschool and school-age children, the presentation by the evaluator of some or all of the following stimulus items may serve to trigger significant fantasizing in the child. The fantasies produced in response to the test items often add further dimension to one's understanding of the child's wishes and fears, his conflicts, and his characteristic ways of coping with stress. The stimulus items listed here can be viewed as semiprojective, much like the items represented in the Rorschach ink blots or in the picture cards of the Thematic Apperception Test (TAT), which a clinical psychologist uses to elicit similar responses.

Often the evaluator has obtained such a wealth of data from the child himself about his background, his feelings, and his everyday functioning that to give the fantasy stimulus items would be redundant. This was certainly the case with Charlie. Accordingly, rather than spending extra time during our second interview on fantasy items that were not really needed to round out my understanding of his conflicts and defenses, I directed Charlie, following a review of the special tests with him, into further discussion of ways he might better handle his angry impulses.

On the other hand, children who are frightened, inhibited, depressed, guarded, or even oppositionally resistive usually have difficulty revealing themselves in the more task-oriented talk of both diagnostic interviews. Such youngsters often require the presentation of many fantasy stimulus items before they begin to share their functioning in greater depth with the interviewer. It sometimes happens that, in addition to eliciting a fantasy response from a child, several of the stimulus items may lead him to begin to share his hopes and fears beyond the given test item—to branch out into a more task-oriented discussion with the interviewer. If that occurs, I generally shift with the child, continuing with as much talk of his own functioning as he is able to engage in for a time. Then, if he stops talking in the area of his daily living, I shift back to the further review of his fantasy life.

Generally, an extensive review of these stimulus items is not necessary with most of the adolescents the evaluator sees. The intensity of adolescents' feelings and their generally good capacity for self-observation go together in creating, in time, an open climate for task-oriented discussions with them. Occasionally, however, presentation of the stimulus items brings a meaningful response from a severely inhibited, depressed, or marginally psychotic teenager that direct questions will not have revealed.

Because the stimulus items were not given to Charlie, another boy's responses serve here to illustrate how a child may
share his fantasy life with us. Alan Mink, a somewhat fragile-
looking six-year-old boy, small for his age, serves as this example. Alan's father, a resident physician at a university hospital, was an intellectually bright but somewhat distant, detached, unaffectionate man. He took pride in his son's growing
academic interests, but did not really feel very close to the
boy, who was an only child. Alan's mother was a chronically
anxious, hand-wringing woman in her early thirties who
seemed obsessed with the idea that Alan would injure himself
in some way. In their initial, joint interview both of them
spelled out the fact that for several years Alan had seemed
to be developing a curious mixture of fearful, cautious, cling-
to-home avoidance behaviors and contradictory bullying-
with-peers, throwing-caution-to-the-winds, slam-bang, aggressive, even assaultive behaviors. As they talked, it became clear
that Alan's often intense and diffuse feelings of apprehension
of impending disaster were beyond normal apprehensions
boys have at this age. Furthermore, it became apparent that
Alan's anxiety remained free-floating in nature, that is, there
was little evidence of definite phobias, conversion reactions,
or obsessive-compulsive symptoms. Indeed, the boy's often
intense anxiety seemed to arise in a variety of situations—even
when, in his parents' judgment, external events around the
boy were calm.

Alan's developmental history was significant in that, from
birth, he was known to have a congenital heart defect. This
was diagnosed in late infancy as a patent ductus arteriosus
with coaractation of the aorta. Because of these defects, Alan
was quite disabled until successful open-heart surgery was
performed when he was two and a half years of age. Although
some cardiomegaly and a mild, persistent right-bundle branch
block were noted by reviewing cardiologists following surgery
and down through the years, these physicians urged the parents to treat their son as a nearly normal child. They were
told to allow him a full range of activities appropriate to his
age; the only injunction was to avoid significant overexertion.
However, to Alan's mother particularly these recommendations seemed aberrant. She was convinced that Alan would
tear his heart open in his play. Accordingly, she watched

closely over him, advising him to go carefully, watch himself, avoid strain, come indoors, not to catch cold, and the like. In these admonitions to her son, Mrs. Mink seemed to the physicians who followed Alan every six months to be unnecessarily infantilizing. Their views, corroborated sharply by emerging signs of Alan's increasingly internalized picture of himself as an overly damaged youngster, led the doctors to recommend that the parents seek evaluation and psychiatric treatment for their son.

In his initial interview with me, Alan was alternately quiet, shy, fearful, and inhibited and loud, boisterous, and devil-may-care. He could say little about his relationships with his parents, teachers, and age-mates or about his chronic handicap, its true extent, and how it affected his feelings and behavior. It was only later, in his second interview with me, that Alan revealed himself more fully through fantasy as the various stimulus items were presented to him.

(1) *Three wishes.* The preschool or school-age child is asked to "play a kind of pretend game. Let's pretend a good fairy wandered in here and could give you any three wishes you wanted to have. I'll count them on my fingers as you tell me what they are." Alan's responses were revealing: (*a*) "I'd want a million dollars. With that I would buy a department store and have all of the guns I wanted. I would also have nail clippers and pocket knives. My mother won't let me have any of these because she says I'll get cut! I would shut out everyone I didn't want to come into my store. On Thursdays I'd hang out a sign that said 'No Women In Here Today!' I would be the one who owned the store and would always win!" (*b*) "To have an elephant" (no further associations). (*c*) "To own a jungle for my elephant" (no further associations).

(2) *A thousand (or a million) dollars.* The child is asked what he feels he might do with this money that he finds "lying in the street." Alan's response led back to his wish for a department store. I recall one anxious, overly inhibited girl of nine with strong superego pressures who said she would immediately "run to the Western Union office to telegraph far and wide the news that the money had been found. Then after that I'd bank the money until its rightful owner came along after hearing the telegram." Another child, an infantilized, indulged, chubby boy of seven, told me: "Oh, boy!

Just think, enough money to buy all the candy in Lexington! And just for me!" As he said this, strings of saliva began to form slowly at the corners of his mouth.

(3) *Animal change*. The child is asked: "Let's pretend you could change yourself into any animal you wanted to be. What would you want to be—and why?" Alan, in responding, became increasingly loud and boisterous. He jumped up from the chair in which he had been sitting, beat his chest with his fists, and cried: "A gorilla! Then I could live all alone in the mountains, not in the city. Then I would play with the other animals, swinging on a rope, and be so strong I could hit anyone in the belly. I could pick up mean people and swing them around or stamp on them. But sometimes I think I'd rather be a mouse instead." When I asked Alan about his mouse idea, he replied; "Well, a mouse—a real tiny one—can't get hurt very much. No one can see him very well and step on him."

(4) *Rocket trip to the moon*. The child is told: "Let's pretend there's a rocket ship that's going to make a trip from down here on earth up to the moon and back. You're the captain. The rocket ship holds two people. Who do you think you'd like to take along with you?" Responding appropriately for a school-age child, Alan said: "I'll take along my best friend, Ricky." Another child, an acutely school-phobic lad of seven, blanched with renewed separation anxiety when I presented this particular stimulus item to him: "Gosh, no! I'm not going there in the first place!"

(5) *Daydream themes*. The evaluator explains to the child using a universalization-generalization approach, that "all kids have daydreams in their heads sometimes. You know, sort of like moving pictures in their heads when they're sitting there at home or at school or anywhere. Their thoughts just sort of drift out the window and go somewhere else. I wonder, I suppose you have daydreams like other boys [or girls]. Can you tell me about a couple of those?" Alan talked, reluctantly at first, and then with increasing anxiety, about sitting in school "thinking about flying saucers. When I hear the police siren outside or an ambulance, it sounds like a flying saucer may have landed. Then I get sorta worried inside because maybe the men from the saucer will come and kidnap the kids in the room. I know it sounds sorta funny, because there really aren't such things as flying saucers. But I think about them

sometimes, anyway." Alan paused. I asked him why he thought
the men from the saucer would want to kidnap children. Near
tears, Alan replied, "Well, you see, they want to start a superior
race of people here on earth. Before they bring their own people here they have to come down and take away all the people
who aren't good ones—who have something wrong with them."
Gently, I asked Alan if, in his daydreams, only other boys and
girls are kidnaped, or if he is taken too. "Oh, it's mostly me
they're after! I've got this big scratch here, you see." Alan
abruptly lifted up his polo shirt to show me the scar across
his chest from the corrective heart surgery. "There's a boy in
school. I hate him! He teases me and says I'll die someday
from this big scratch!" Open tears now. "I chase him and
knock him down and grind his face! He can't say things like
that to me! It isn't true." From this point, with further support from me, Alan went on to describe, in a whining, scowl-
ing, complaining manner, that "Mom and Dad won't let me
do a lot of things. Especially my mother. She won't let me
play rough, or go to the basement, or play ball in the park.
She's afraid I'll get hurt. My mother won't let me do anything."

(6) *Night dream themes.* Generally, I explain to children
that "dreams at night are sometimes friendly ones. And sometimes they're not so friendly, sort of scary dreams. Everybody
has some friendly dreams and some scary ones, too. Can you
tell me about a friendly dream you've had? And a scary one?"
Some children, even with this support, cannot recall a specific
dream of their own. One can then say something like: "Well,
okay, all of us can't remember our dreams sometimes. But
what would be your best guess about a scary dream a boy of
your age might have?" The child often goes on then to make
up a fantasied dream embodying his own concerns. Alan, however, responded directly to the stimulus item. "I get this scary
dream over and over again of big monsters coming into my
room and chewing on my chest!" Recurrent dreams like this
are often an indicator of significant underlying conflict.

Often such a nightmare is a potent mixture, as in Alan's
case, of a rather direct expression of the child's overreactive
concerns about his own bodily functioning and his identification with the aggressor. In his dream, Alan at one and the
same time is the victim of heart surgery and surgeons and the

monster himself, who does to others what they do to him. In this latter role, Alan is no longer the helpless, passive recipient of bodily experiences too large for him to meet and master, but becomes the active doer instead—the one who turns the tables on others. This turning of passivity into activity, often through the mechanism of identification with the aggressor, is a fairly common coping technique children use to handle underlying fears in fantasies of all types.

(7) *The Despert Fables* (see Appendix for a full listing). In arranging a series of incomplete stories that embody developmental tasks and the natural anxieties over growth that accompany them, Louise Despert some years ago furnished us with another frequently useful stimulus list for children's fantasies.[9] Generally, each story is told to the child from the evaluator's memory, or each story is read to him from a printed list. The child's response to the stories is elicited in the following manner: "I'm going to read you some stories. Each one needs an ending. I'd like you to tell me how you think each story ends."

Alan's responses to a major portion of the Despert Fables paralleled his other fantasy responses. (*a*) *Bird Fable*: "Both the mother bird and the father bird fly down and bring the baby bird back to the nest. They tell him he won't be ready to fly for a long time." (*b*) *Lamb Fable*: "The big one is glad and eats grass. Gee, just think—he gets to run around all over that field while the mother sheep is tied up with the baby lamb!" (*c*) *Elephant Fable*: "The elephant's trunk is all torn up and bleeding" (Alan was anxiously restive as he responded). "I don't know what happened to it. Or how it happened. Must have been something pretty awful, though!" (*d*) *Anxiety Fable*: "I don't know what the boy is worried about. Maybe about getting sick sometimes and not being able to do things." (*e*) *Funeral Fable:* "An old man died. Not sure who. Or why." (*f*) *Good News Fable*: "The boy heard that his birthday is coming and he is going to have a real big party!" (Alan was grinning somewhat as he responded.) (*g*) *Bad News Fable*: "He can't go out and play. He got sick and his mother won't let him play." At this point, Alan referred again to his own open-heart surgery scar, which he called his "big scratch."

9. "Despert Fables," *American Journal of Orthopsychiatry, 16*, January 1946, pp. 100-13.

Just then, encouraged by Alan's having shared some disturbed feelings over several fantasy-stimulus items, we were able to shift to a more revealing, feeling-oriented discussion in which several things came to light: Alan's doubts about his own present and future functioning; his distortions of his body image—he wasn't really certain what his heart did, what had been wrong with it in the first place, and what surgery had been performed on it; and, finally, his questions about the exercise he could have now in the judgment of his primary physician. Alan's doubts about himself responded somewhat to the rough diagrams I drew for him, accompanied by simple explanations of cardiac functions, the true nature of his past handicap, what surgery was performed, and my understanding of what he could and could not do at this point in his life and in the future.

In this way, *the interviewer sometimes has an opportunity to begin therapeutic discussion with a child in the midst of evaluation interviews* whose main purpose is the gathering of data that point up the child's conflicts and defenses. Children do not wait for evaluation interviews to end before they begin exploring their hopes and fears. Sometimes, like Alan Mink, they move back and forth in their talks with us between saying or showing something about themselves in a diagnostic way and raising feeling-oriented opportunities for us to respond in a therapeutic direction. This tendency might be defined as moments having therapeutic potential that can come during any diagnostic interview with a child.

(8) *Free play and structured play sequences.* As Robert Waelder indicated some years ago, children's free play can often be viewed as fantasy woven around play objects.[10] Erik H. Erikson carried this theme forward when he postulated that play can frequently be taken as the child's attempts to master, in model form, the normal developmental anxieties that attend the crucial tasks posed by succeeding stages of development.[11] Viewed this way, the endless games of mothers-and-fathers played out by preschool boys and girls, to cite only one example, give these children opportunities to practice appropriate gender role behavior about which they are becoming increasingly cognizant. In our diagnostic interviews with

10. "The Psychoanalytic Theory of Play," *Zeitschrift für Psychoanalytische Padogogik* VI, 1932.
11. *Childhood and Society*, 211.

children, moreover, these same considerations shape our conclusions about the meaning of children's play with materials in the playroom. Here, too, are examples of fantasies woven about play objects.

Free play is that which the child chooses for himself. Structured play involves some initial ordering of play events by the evaluator, who asks the child, for example, to "pick a family" from among a variety of flexible rubber dolls and have it go through a number of potentially conflictual and nonconflictual situations.

Many are the varieties of free and structured play themes that might be constructed either by the child or by the evaluator. The kinds of play are shaped by the presenting problems in the child himself and by the evaluator's own creativity. The general difficulty I encounter in using free or structured play to obtain fantasy material from a child is finding enough time. Two separate diagnostic interviews with each child are already crowded with discussions, special tests, and the other, more rapidly applied stimulus items used to produce fantasy responses in children. Besides, a child who has been helped to settle into his interviews and is revealing himself quite well in these other ways does not need play as such to reveal himself further. Instead, as was said in an earlier chapter, free and structured play techniques can be reserved for the fearful, inhibited, overly anxious, or depressed child who cannot, in a reasonable time, be helped to use talking as a predominant mode of communication. For such children play materials may well be needed to open up communication, but for most others they are rarely required.

THE PHYSICAL AND NEUROLOGICAL EXAMINATIONS

We turn now to another basic part of the diagnostic process, the appraisal of a child's physical and neurological status. In the physical area, this includes an evaluation of data from both the developmental history and the general physical examination, as well as any special studies that might have been required in the past. Although these physical studies have usually been made before the troubled child is referred for evaluation, the evaluator must acquaint himself with their extent, adequacy, and current status. If the evaluator is a physician, he can telephone or write the primary physician for a brief report of the child's physical status. If he is not, however, he must ask a physician who works with him—the medical director of a clinic, for example—to correspond directly with the child's primary physician to obtain the needed information.

Sometimes the evaluator of the troubled child must gauge the need for further physical studies. These would be required, for example, when a primary physician who overemphasizes emotional factors refers a child without having carefully assessed the child's somatic status. And when children are referred from nonmedical sources, it is the responsibility of the physician-evaluator, or a physician working in collaboration with him, to plan for reliable physical examination. In clinics or in private practice, psychiatrists and other evaluators should have good working arrangements for obtaining physical studies by competent physicians. The psychiatrist usually does not perform the general physical examination of the child himself; it is done on referral to someone else.

The situation may be different with regard to the neurological examinations. Many psychiatrists are both willing and able to perform such examinations on children whom they or their colleagues are evaluating whenever the need arises. Those who do not wish to conduct neurological examinations, however, will refer children to a reliable neurologist to complete a developmentally oriented study.

For psychiatrists in training who may desire to conduct their own neurological examinations of children, under appropriate supervision by a teaching neurologist, a useful model is given at the end of this book (see Appendix). The outline set down here is one I have adapted for my occasional use from a model developed some years ago by Dr. Abraham Wikler, Professor of Psychiatry, and Dr. Robert Aug, Professor of Child Psychiatry and Director of the Division of Child Psychiatry at the University of Kentucky College of Medicine. Their outline makes provision for the fact that relatively minor deviations in a child's basic somatic equipment, such as mild visual or auditory disturbances, are no less significant than gross physical handicaps and neurological disorders in their potential effect on the child's adaptive capacities. Disorders of perception and poor motor coordination may seriously interfere with the child's ability to meet educational and social challenges. Such disorders may occur in a variety of psychiatric disturbances, including brain injury.

The diagnosis of minimal disturbances of central nervous system functions may be very difficult. Often careful observation of the child in his playroom activities during his other interviews, with special emphasis on his neurophysiological patterns, is more significant diagnostically than the more formal and classical neurological examination. As an example, Charlie's interview behavior during our two sessions together clearly showed him to be a healthy child with no signs of neuromuscular abnormality. For Charlie, then, no neurological examination was needed. The same conclusion holds true for many troubled children referred for diagnostic evaluation.

But for those like nine-year-old Billy (mentioned earlier in this chapter) whose behavior and performance on the special screening tests clearly suggest a perceptual-visual-motor problem or other neuromuscular abnormality, it is imperative that the physician-evaluator either refer the child to a neurologist for an evaluation or perform the needed neurological examination himself. For the occasional child whom I examine myself, I arrange a special third appointment. As outlined in the Appendix, this examination is time-consuming, requiring upwards of an hour and a half to complete even with the most cooperative child. Children's attention spans and, accordingly, their ability to cooperate naturally lag if appointments are prolonged into several hours. For this reason, it is better to have the child return refreshed, on a different day, for a third appointment for the neurological examination.

In Billy's case, my neurological review indicated that a number of soft, or equivocal, neurological signs were present. Most noticeable were ataxia and difficulty with postural equilibrium on tandem walking, toe walking, heel walking, and hopping in place on one foot. The difficulty with postural equilibrium was also clearly noticeable while standing on one foot, and while standing with eyes closed and arms elevated forward. Postural disequilibrium was not noticed while Billy stood with his arms down at his sides. The boy showed past-pointing on finger-to-nose and finger-to-finger movements. Extraneous movements and clowning, as if to cover disability and/or anxiety, were frequently present, especially during the parts of the examination where Billy had difficulty. On the sensory side, the only abnormal finding was marked impairment of graphesthesia. In tests of lateral dominance, Billy's reports and those of others indicated mixed dominance, and I had noted this during the earlier two interviews. However, during the formal neurological examination, his dominance remained essentially on the right. His ocular dominance seemed to be left. Regarding right-left orientation, Billy showed intermittent confusion during early trials, but he improved later.

These neurological findings on Billy, when put alongside his problems in reading and his problems in perceptual-visual-motor functioning picked up on the previous special screening tests, clearly suggested that he might have some degree of minimal brain dysfunction. To further define the degree of this impairment, it was necessary at that point to have Billy tested by a clinical psychologist.

When I raised this need for further psychological testing with Billy's parents, they were quite willing to accept the additional procedure as an aid to the overall evaluation of the boy's limitations and assets. To help prepare Billy for the testing, I explained the purpose of the tests to him and, at the time of his appointment for testing in the clinic, introduced him to the clinical psychologist with whom he would be meeting for several testing sessions.

THE PSYCHOLOGICAL EXAMINATION

Psychological testing is particularly indicated when the primary evaluator of the child feels that screening data suggest the existence of specific learning disabilities, mental retardation, the possibility of chronic brain injury, or the existence of borderline or actual psychosis. Such testing thus has the additional function of helping to obtain a general picture of the child's problem areas and defenses.

In most clinics, several types of psychological tests are generally used—intelligence tests, achievement tests, projective tests, and special techniques such as tests for brain damage. The Stanford-Binet and the Wechsler Intelligence Scale for Children (for children age six and older) and the Wechsler Adult Scale (for adolescents) are given as intelligence tests. A Binet test is available for preschool children down to the age of two years, and other tests, such as the Psyche Cattell Infant Tests, the Bailey Scales for Infant Development, the Gesell Scale of Development, and the Merrill-Palmer Scales have been devised for infants and preschool children. The reliability of infants' and very young children's tests is comparatively poor in and of themselves, exclusive of other studies of the child. In general, it can be said that a high score on a test has more significance and validity than a low score. These tests are often helpful, however, in making gross distinctions between very bright and very dull intelligences. The reliability of any intelligence test score for a child under the age of four or five is open to question.

Although performance on an intelligence test is certainly vulnerable to anxiety and emotional upset, the test often (but not necessarily) gives a better picture than projective tests of the child's assets and what he can do best. When it does so, it is because the intelligence test is structured and, by the time the child is of school age, the procedure of tapping his knowledge and intellectual functioning is somewhat familiar to him. Unless he is undergoing acute anxiety about the testing situation, in which case he should not be tested at that time, the intelligence test performance yields the more valid insights into the child's capabilities, be they meager or abundant.

Achievement tests, such as the Wide Range Achievement Tests (WRAT), measure the benefits the child has derived from his educational endeavors and cultural background. Often the lack of correlation between educational achievement and mental ability uncovers the nature of learning problems (whether general or specific, such as in reading or arithmetic) or points up cultural deprivation in a particular child.

Projective tests have in common the presentation of relatively unstructured material to the child so that his responses are more a function of his subjective reactions and his internal dynamics than of the test material. Nonetheless, projective tests differ in the degree of structuring they present, and this difference is important in evaluating performance results. Children differ in their ability to tolerate unfamiliarity and lack of structure, but in general these conditions tend to arouse a certain amount of anxiety and hostility. Many responses to projective tests are a reflection of the child's conflicts or his defenses against them. Moreover, such tests permit responses which are of a more primitive and impulse-ridden nature than responses to more structured tests. Thus the projective variety tend to stress the conflicts within the child but do not always indicate the clinical significance of the apparent psychopathology. This does not mean that such assets as creativity and ego strengths are not tapped by these tests, but that care must be used to avoid overestimating the degree of psychopathology.

Among the projective tests, the Rorschach ink-blot technique is the most unstructured and often the one most likely to reveal nuclear conflicts, basic anxieties, and the level of emotional maturation. The Rorschach scoring categories do provide some insight into personality functioning inasmuch as the sharpness of reality testing, the nature of the ego defenses, the degree of anxiety, and the capacity for emotional control and inner life are among the many aspects of personality structure which can be evaluated. Tests like the Thematic Apperception Test, the Children's Apperception Test, and the Michigan Picture Test, where the child is asked to tell stories in response to pictures, are more structured; they apparently reveal less of the child's instinctual conflicts than the Rorschach technique, and therefore they sometimes give a better balanced picture of the child's ego weaknesses and strengths. These picture-story methods focus on the child's defenses or ways of handling interpersonal and social situations; they reveal what he perceives as being the major internal and external forces acting on him and his methods of meeting these needs and forces. The Draw-a-Person test, which is considered a reflection of the child's body-image, gives some insight into the child's self-image.

Projective tests, by their nature, are generally more reliable for school-age children, whose personalities are more structured, than for preschool children. The different facets of personality which these projective measures tap and the different degrees of pathology they measure point to the need for a battery of tests in order to obtain a well-rounded personality picture. Thus an intelligence test and a variety of projective tests are necessary to arrive at a useful personality description.

The test battery becomes important, too, in attempting to evaluate brain injury in children. The WISC or the Binet test may provide data indicating that the child has specific impairments in intellectual functioning, such as numerical reasoning, verbal abstraction, the immediate recording and manipulation of the memory trace, remote memory, or the ability to deal with commonsense problems. The Bender Visual-Motor Gestalt Test and the Graham-Kendall Memory for Design Test, which involve the child's copying geometric figures, may provide clues suggesting that he has specific impairments in perceptual-visual-motor functioning; these are suspected if the organization of these test figures and their forms are destroyed when the child copies them. Organic brain impairment may be reflected on the Rorschach by the appearance of a significant number of signs of this condition; namely, one may detect an inability to handle color, or the repetition of certain responses. None of these test signs by itself is a positive indicator (the clinical history and the child's performance on the neurological examination must also be taken into account), and, in fact, diagnosis of brain injury cannot be made on the basis of these psychological tests alone. Nevertheless, if provided with sufficient data a skilled psychologist can often pick up enough indications from a battery of psychological tests to suggest the possibility of brain damage.

The validity of projective test results is highly dependent on the skill, the experience, and the personality of the psychologist and the kind of relationship that has been set up between the child and the tester. This dependence does not invalidate the test results as long as the tester is sensitive to these effects. Test interpretation is enhanced by this sensitivity on the part of the examiner, but when the sensitivity is lacking, test results may be distorted.

Psychological examinations, like physical and neurological examinations, are not ends in themselves. Rather, all three areas of inquiry are aids to the evaluator, the child's parents, and the child himself in their fuller understanding of the child's assets and liabilities—a necessary first step in their joint endeavor to find ways and means of resolving difficulties. Most frequently, psychological test results are used by the evaluator as another source of information to guide him in dealing further with the parents and child.

In the final chapter of this book we examine the way the evaluator pulls together, or sums up, all these varied types of information about a child into a comprehensive formulation of the child's problems and assets. And we see how the evaluator does this in a way most meaningful to the child's parents as he meets with them in the follow-up conference that concludes the diagnostic evaluation. But before we turn to that important final part of the diagnostic study, we need to consider certain other areas of review that occasionally provide us with important additional data; Chapter 9 discusses some elective procedures that may prove valuable to the evaluator.

Chapter 9.

Elective Procedures in the Evaluation

Occasionally, during the course of a comprehensive study of a particular child, the evaluator may find himself in a real diagnostic dilemma. He may feel that some critically important data are missing, data that would enable him to understand fully the daily functioning of the child. It is not that he, the parents, and the child have not tried to supply, or uncover, the missing pieces in the diagnostic jigsaw puzzle as they have met together. It seems rather that certain factors have obscured the needed information instead of revealing it. Sometimes these factors lie in the feelings and attitudes of the child's parents; sometimes they are part of the child's own feelings, blocking him from revealing himself fully in office interviews. In either case, the methods, procedures, and techniques described earlier in this book have not been successful in facilitating the forward flow of the interviews with the family. The evaluator is left very much in the dark, wondering how the family really functions outside his office.

If this should happen—and, fortunately, such occurrences are rare—the evaluator may resort to several additional diagnostic "aces up his sleeve" described in this chapter. Here again, stories about specific children for whom such elective procedures were required are used to illustrate the following discussion of these techniques.

PROCEDURES CLARIFYING THE DEVELOPMENTAL
HISTORY OF THE CHILD

The use of the developmental questionnaire is not always

effective. The parents may literally have forgotten some very important early-life data about their child. For the majority of children one sees in evaluation, however, this is not a critical matter. After all, most of us adults quite naturally have difficulty recalling many of the details of our own children's growth with the passage of years. The parents of the children we see can be expected to do no better or no worse than we in compiling retrospective data on their children.

But for certain children the parents' inability to recall large blocks of data, through repression or denial, can be a critical matter. For example, if one is evaluating a preschool child who is mute and has significant difficulty in relating with other people, the diagnostic picture is clarified by detailed knowledge of the child's developmental background. In such a case, one would consider the possibility that the child was totally or partially deaf, or had some form of aphasic disturbance, or was mentally retarded, or had an autistic psychosis of early childhood. The differential diagnosis would depend primarily on the evaluator's detailed observation of such a child's behavior coupled with the parents' account of the child's functioning at home. Special tests, such as clinical psychological testing and audiometry, would supplement these other data in important ways. But still, a detailed knowledge of the child's milestones in growth through the years would be of great assistance in the total evaluation.

Some years ago I encountered just such a problem in making a differential diagnosis. This was in the case of Carrie Hammersmith, a well-developed, dark-haired, brown-eyed girl of six whom we met in Chapter 5. The reader will recall that Carrie was relatively mute and did not relate with people at all. Instead, in her evaluation interviews she related intensely—with highly detailed performance skills—to things like plastic building sets, puzzles, and form-boards.

Carrie's parents were remarkably alike in being relatively cold, detached, mechanistic, compulsive persons who had great difficulty expressing themselves emotionally to each other and to Carrie, their only child. In their joint and their separate interviews with me, this affectionless quality was quite striking. They seemed to be using isolation of affect as a defense against the anxiety caused by living together. Indeed, each seemed to exist in a private world of activities, leaving the three family members under one roof but quite apart from one another. Carrie, of course, seemed wrapped away in deafness, aphasia, or autism. Jim Hammersmith, thirty-two, was preoccupied with his hobby of photography. Carrie's mother, Elizabeth, thirty, seemed largely to divide her time at home between housecleaning and the study of brochures on furs. She was the head buyer of furs for a department store in their community.

It was not too difficult for Jim and Elizabeth Hammersmith to describe Carrie's current day-to-day functioning to me. From what they said, I obtained no indication that Carrie was deaf. In her jargon speech, in fact, she sometimes carefully imitated the rubbing of insect wings, the rustle of leaves, and the sounds of some animals. (Later, clinical audiometry substantiated these interview impressions of Carrie's receptive and spoken language usage in certain areas.) Instead, what her parents described to me of Carrie's current behavior suggested that she was an autistic child.

But what was missing in their description of their daughter was their recall of anything significant about Carrie's growth from birth to about five years of age. This rather massive forgetting, by both of them, became evident when Mrs. Hammersmith brought in the developmental questionnaire she and her husband were to have filled out together. Beyond putting down identifying information about family members on the face sheet of the questionnaire, the couple had supplied nothing else that would help me trace Carrie's development as a probably autistic child. Mrs. Hammersmith said both she and her husband had spent considerable time attempting to fill out the form. Finally, however, they had abandoned the task when it became apparent that neither could recall the data asked for.

Developmental Data. At this point, still desiring to have developmental data on Carrie's growth, I asked Mrs. Hammersmith if the couple had kept records of any type about the child. She looked puzzled for a moment. Then she mentioned that although her husband had spent no time holding, bathing, feeding, or playing with Carrie, he seemed to have enjoyed taking a great many pictures of their daughter as she grew up. These pictures had been preserved in a number of albums. This seemed promising, and I set another individual appointment for Mrs. Hammersmith, asking her to bring in all of these albums.

She appeared at the next interview with a stack of seven albums. There were pictures of Carrie engaged in all sorts of impersonal activities. Jim Hammersmith had taken pictures of his daughter almost every month of her six years. Mrs. Hammersmith, for her part, had been meticulous in dating and captioning each picture.

These pictures proved to be helpful, indeed; some important stages of Carrie's development were depicted clearly. In addition, with the aid of the photographs Mrs. Hammersmith was able, at certain points, to recall some of the details of the events her husband had photographed. For example, one photograph, labeled "Carrie—four months," showed the child sitting upright in a bouncy-chair in their kitchen. Another photograph was of Carrie standing up, at seven months of age, holding on to the coffee table for support. Still another picture showed the child, then twelve months old, walking about on her own without support or assistance. From these pictures it was apparent that Carrie had met and mastered the major milestones of motor development at the same times in her infancy as most of her peers. Another set of pictures, which Mrs. Hammersmith had labeled as taken during Carrie's third and fourth years, were of the child coloring with crayons on paper and finger-painting. There were, as well, photographs of some of these productions themselves. One drawing, captioned "Carrie, three years and seven months, crayon-on-paper," was a series of perfectly formed circles connected by curving lines. Carrie had colored each of the circles a different color. Her work was quite meticulous. She had colored each circle completely, yet had stayed within the lines she had drawn for them. Another drawing, dated a year later, was much more complex. It consisted of a variety of rather geometric shapes—circles, squares, lines, and triangles—assembled in a free-form design.

From these rather detailed performance aspects of her drawings, and from the fact that her motor-muscular development was typical for a child her age, I drew the conclusion that Carrie was probably not an intellectually retarded child. Later, of course, in her office interviews Carrie showed exceptional performance skills in working with clay and play dough and in making intricate constructions with blocks and the plastic building set. There again, her performance skills were actually advanced for a six-year-old child.

Releasing Feelings. But our review together of the picture albums uncovered another—and perhaps the most vital—area of the family's functioning. To be sure, I had gained important data and impressions about some aspects of Carrie's early development. But, beyond this, as she began to recall more and more about Carrie's growth as we looked at and discussed the pictures together, Mrs. Hammersmith began to reveal some feelings as well. I was particularly struck, as we looked at pictures her husband had taken of Carrie as an infant, by this woman's genuine puzzlement and confusion. One picture showed Carrie drinking milk from a bottle that was propped up on a rolled pillow in her crib. As she looked at this photograph, Mrs. Hammersmith seemed quite confused for a moment. When I reflected that I noticed what looked like bewilderment in her face, she came almost to tears. Her statements then, for the first time in our interviews, revealed how troubled this mother had been all along with this mute, impersonal, strange, yet intelligent child.

"Oh, Dr. Looff, I just remembered there for a minute how hard it was for me with Carrie. It started when I was pregnant with her. I mean, I was really scared! I got this awful feeling I would never be any good for my child. I would sit there, before the child was born, for hours, feeling sort of, well, frozen up inside. Oh, I couldn't say anything about my feelings to Jim. He doesn't listen, and feelings of any kind trouble him. So I said nothing. But after Carrie was born this freezing-up inside me was even stronger. Maybe it was there because I was an only child and didn't really know what to expect with a new baby. Maybe not. Anyway, I stayed scared most of the time. And Carrie was so funny-acting. Like she never wanted to be touched. I'd try, if I wasn't feeling so frozen up, to hold her to feed her. But she'd stiffen up like a board. It got so I didn't ever want to hold her. It made me feel like I was right all along—no good as a mother. So that's why the bottle was given to her the way you see in this picture. It was easier for me, and for Carrie, too, I guess, to feed her this way."

On further questioning about Carrie's infancy, Mrs. Hammersmith was then able to say that the child had never developed the milestones in her emotional development typical of a child engaged in a normal, need-satisfying mother-child relationship. For example, Carrie rarely established eye contact with her mother—during feeding or at any other time. The following response in her was not established at two months of age and thereafter. Unlike most infants at four months of age and older, Carrie did not smile on seeing her parents' faces nor did she, then or ever throughout her infancy, assume an anticipatory posture (grin, outstretched arms) when she was picked up. "It looked like she didn't know us, or something. No, I didn't discuss this with our pediatrician. I guess I hoped that it was just me, and we'd get along better as she grew up. But I did wonder, when she didn't talk and continued to treat us as though we weren't ever there, if something was wrong. I thought at first she was deaf, and so did Jim. When she was four we talked with our doctor about Carrie. He sent us to the Speech and Hearing Center here in town. After they studied her for six months, they said she was not deaf, and that the problem was an emotional one."

Through the use of the picture albums, then, I had learned something more about Carrie's development in the motor-muscular, speech, intellectual-cognitive, interpersonal, and social areas. Important, too, was the fact that this pictured approach to their daughter's growth aided Mrs. Hammersmith to recall more historical data and also to start recalling and experiencing feelings from the past that had probably shaped her mothering role with Carrie. In so doing, she had revealed a pattern rather typical of parents whose children are later diagnosed as being autistic. For congenital, biological reasons as yet unclear to us as clinicians (the British, notably among them Michael Rutter,[1] believe this organic substrate of autism is a language-coding problem), the child is not capable as an infant of responding to his parents' approaches. Often, too, at least one of the parents (or both, as with the Hammersmiths) is a rather remote, compulsive, repressed, and inhibited individual. Because of these personality traits, such people are unsure of themselves in the parenting role. The child's

1. "Intelligence and Childhood Psychiatric Disorder," *British Journal of Social and Clinical Psychology*, 3, 1964, pp. 120-29.

failure to react is interpreted by them as proof that they are, indeed, poor mothers and fathers, and consequently they withdraw even further from their developing child. For his part, the latter gradually withdraws into a private world of intense preoccupation with things, a world in which people are excluded.

This picture approach to Carrie's development was something I attempted with Jim Hammersmith as well. Although he was mildly pleased with my comments about his excellent pictures of Carrie, he could not recall much further information or share his inner feelings with me as his wife had done. Throughout our conversation, in effect, he seemed to be a remote, cold, distance-promoting, rather affectionless man. However, he did share a further historical recording of one important aspect of an autistic child's functioning. I refer here to what Leo Kanner described years ago as the autistic child's intense preoccupation with sameness.[2] These children, exclusively preoccupied with their intricate manipulation of things in their environment, are driven into anxiety states of panic proportions if people interfere in some manner with their preoccupation with whatever it is they are doing at the moment.

When I asked Jim Hammersmith whether he recalled Carrie's ever having shown such behavior, he finally remembered that these states occurred occasionally. And he remembered that he had recorded one such episode on home-movie film. At my request, he brought this film and his projector to my office for review during a later interview.

The filmed sequence was taken in their home. On this particular occasion, Carrie's mother had taken a bowl of plastic fruit that formed the centerpiece for their dining-room table to the kitchen. There she had washed the fruit and placed it on the drainboard to dry. Several hours later she replaced the fruit in the bowl, which she put back on the table—all except a pineapple, which she left on the drainboard to dry further. Carrie apparently came into the kitchen and saw the lone pineapple there. Later, when her mother put the pineapple into the bowl with the other fruit, Carrie removed it and placed it back on the kitchen drainboard where she had

2. *Child Psychiatry* (Springfield, Ill.: Charles C. Thomas, 1935).

initially seen it. Mr. Hammersmith began filming the struggle between Carrie and her mother over the pineapple. At first to both parents it seemed "cute." Mrs. Hammersmith would take the pineapple from the kitchen to the bowl on the dining-room table. Carrie, in a moment or two, would check the bowl, remove only the pineapple, and march it back to the drain-board. This behavior continued for several filmed sequences. Then, while Mr. Hammersmith filmed the moment, Mrs. Hammersmith remained in the dining room and prevented Carrie from removing the pineapple a fourth time by holding her hand on the fruit in the bowl. In the film, Carrie looked puzzled for a moment. She attempted to move her mother's hand from the fruit in a mechanical, derrick-like manner. Her mother resisted this. Then Carrie began what appeared to be a frenzied, screaming, foot-stamping, hair-pulling, dress-tearing moment of panic, and her startled mother could not console her (Mr. Hammersmith stopped filming to attempt to assist his wife). The episode apparently terminated just as spontane-ously as it had erupted, a few minutes later. Thus, in the home-movie film, I had seen a typical example of an autistic child's intense preoccupation with sameness.

From these experiences with Carrie and her parents, I drew the conclusion that picture albums, baby books, and even home movies can at times be useful supplements to the devel-opmental questionnaire and to discussions the evaluator has with parents about the early development of their child. These methods or techniques, as I have indicated here, are not usually required in the course of an evaluation. But for repressed, in-hibited, remote, nonrecalling parents these methods may ef-fectively uncork developmental data and feelings as well—both crucial in the establishment of a therapeutic alliance with parents.

HOME VISITS

In the discussion of interview settings in Chapter 3, the point was made that occasionally the evaluator may elect to see a child in his home setting for one, or even all, of his evaluation interviews. Timothy Sizemore was given as an example of severely frightened, inhibited, or depressed children who often do not relate well at first with the strange evaluator in his office. The reader will recall how miserable and essentially non-talkative the severely inhibited Tim was with me during that first interview hour in the clinic. I felt that I could not at that point draw any really valid conclusions about his functioning as a person beyond what I had learned of his fright and personality inhibition. It was obvious that I would have to see him further in a setting more familiar to him if both his problems and any strengths he might possess were to be properly assessed. Accordingly, I elected to visit Tim at his home for our next interview. That meeting succeeded in enabling a relationship to begin so that Tim could eventually tell me of his troubled feelings and share with me some of his hopes and plans.

Some acutely school-phobic younger children often literally force us out of our offices; we have to begin seeing them at home. Through the spreading phenomenon fairly typical of all phobic reactions, these children sometimes develop a clinic phobia as well. They can no more separate from home to meet the evaluator in his office than they can leave home to attend school. The frustrated parents then tell the evaluator—by telephone, or in the office where they have come without the child—that they are powerless to bring their child in to see him. In such a case, the evaluator may elect to go to the child at home to begin their meeting and talking there. Over the past twelve years, I have had many occasions to meet acutely school- and clinic-phobic children from the hills of Eastern Kentucky at their homes. And often, as we've met and talked in barnyards, in gardens, and on cabin front porches, or while walking woodland trails together, the children and I have discovered that such home visits have been effective in reducing fears sufficiently for them to be able subsequently to meet with me in my field clinic in the local health departments. These examples point up how home visits are almost a matter of necessity early in the evaluation and treatment of some children.

There is, moreover, another use of home visits that, in a sense, is more elective than in the instances cited above. There are a few cases where the child has no difficulty at all coming to the office for evaluation, or separating from his parents to meet with the evaluator alone, and yet the nature of his problems, his accustomed ways of coping with stress, and his ego strengths still remain obscure after a number of office talks. With these children the advantage of home visits is that there, in their natural habitats, they often reveal themselves more fully and clear up earlier mysteries.

I recall, for example, one particular five-and-a-half-year-old boy, Ricky Swartz, whose parents brought him for evaluation several years ago. As it turned out, the life-styles of Ricky's parents, their distancing each other in their marriage, and their inability to relate very well with their son except along intellectual lines remarkably paralleled the functioning of the family of Peter Schlatz, mentioned in Chapter 8. Like Peter, Ricky in his two evaluation interviews with me related very poorly. His fantasies revealed significant disturbance in reality testing and intense preoccupation with personal injury at the hands of overpowering adults. Just as I concluded about Peter, I gained the clinical impression that Ricky was growing up to be a borderline psychotic child.

Thus my clinical impressions about Ricky, built up on office interview data, were sufficient to establish a working diagnosis of the boy's problems. But I did not really know, near the end of that collaborative diagnostic study, what relationship strengths or what other skills Ricky might possess. My collaborator, Billy Ables, a clinical psychologist, had been unable, because of the considerable extent to which the parents used denial, to engage the couple in a feeling-oriented exchange of data about the boy. Mrs. Swartz, particularly, covered all her stories about Ricky with denial of almost saccharine quality. She smiled literally over everything. In this way her real feelings about herself, her marriage, and the behavior of this strange but intellectually bright little boy were hidden from herself, from her husband, from Ricky, and now from Dr. Ables. Near the end of our collaborative study of the family, as Dr. Ables and I discussed it together, we felt that we had all the data needed to make a diagnosis. But we lacked interview knowledge of the boy's basic relationship skills at their best (in my hours with Ricky he avoided eye contact altogether and spent his time staying away from me by playing over toys, mumbling near-psychotic fantasied stories as he played). And we lacked any interview knowledge of whether or not Mrs. Swartz could be reached vis-à-vis her true feelings. These were important points to be determined if we were to recommend outpatient care for the family as opposed to residential, inpatient treatment for the youngster.

Searching for Further Skills and Feelings. Accordingly, Dr. Ables and I decided that I would visit Ricky in his home in an effort to clarify these two critical points. Although she seemed somewhat puzzled by our request, Mrs. Swartz nonetheless agreed to my meeting their son there. The home visit was timed for the hour between two and three o'clock one particular afternoon. I would have the opportunity to meet them when Mrs. Swartz and Ricky were home alone during that time. And, near the end of the visit, I could expect to see how the boy interacted with his eight-year-old sister, Kathy, who would be returning from her day in her second-grade class.

The two-story, traditional brick home belonging to the Swartzes was located on a curving drive in a new, upper-middle-class suburb of Lexington. When they were transferred from New York a year prior to coming to the clinic, the couple had purchased this home from the previous owner for a substantial sum. Mrs. Swartz had earlier indicated that her husband's salary as a certified public accountant at the local plant of a national firm enabled them to keep up the payments on their home without too much difficulty. She told Dr. Ables, "Everyone adores the house! Why, Kathy has expressed a wish my husband and I get out of it in later years, transfer on I guess she means, so she can live in it all alone when she is older." (When Mrs. Swartz made this comment, Dr. Ables, who was beginning to see Kathy as the most mature member of the family, thought to herself that these comments might be more nearly an expression of Kathy's wish to be rid of her parents and her brother than the "adoring" interpretation Mrs. Swartz had placed upon them.)

At the time of my visit, Mrs. Swartz met me effusively at the front door. Her words and tones carried the saccharine quality that marked her talking in the clinic. But that afternoon, as she pointed out that she had "lighted a nice, cheery fire on our hearth to warm your visit and this gray day," there was the beginning of an anxiety-determined rattle to Mrs.

Swartz's voice. Some tension was beginning to show through, I felt. Continuing, she said, "You go right on and make yourself comfortable—just make yourself at home. Ricky is preoccupied in the basement with the two men who are putting in the new water softener down there. So I guess you'll find him there. I'm just going to go on about my business here in the kitchen and pretend that you're not here at all!" It was obvious that my coming had triggered some anxiety in her. I thanked her, making a few comments about the tasteful furnishings of their home. She smiled, rather thinly I felt, and showed me the door leading to the basement stairs.

In the basement, Ricky was playing off by himself in a playroom corner. He was not watching the two men who were clattering and banging on pipes just twelve feet from where he sat on the floor. The boy looked up at my approach, briefly established eye contact with me, smiled slightly, and said: "You're Dr. Looff." Then he dropped his gaze and returned to his self-absorbed interest in taking apart and accurately reassembling a plastic toy he told me was "a panic button." At this point, although Ricky had interacted briefly with me, more interest was directed my way from the others there. The two men kept watching me, in an obvious attempt to figure out who I was and what I was doing there. And the family's toy French poodle, Maurice, frantically and joyfully scampered about my legs, jumped up, and responded positively to my patting him. In an attempt to reach the boy by extending my natural interaction with the poodle to him, I asked Ricky his dog's name. He did not look up as he replied, simply, "Maurice." He continued to take apart the toy with which he had ostensibly been so absorbed. In about ten minutes the workmen, their task completed, packed up their tool boxes, exchanged a few words with me, and departed.

At this point, Ricky went over to the new water-conditioner tank, examined it carefully, and began to open the fuse box controlling the electrical wiring leading to it. I followed him. He looked at me and asked: "Is this the electricity box that goes to the new water conditioner? Will you open it? Please open it!" I told him he had figured out the box correctly, but that it would be unsafe to play with the fuse box. "Could we play together with something else, instead?" I asked. The boy turned away and got out some plastic bowling pins and a ball from a toybox. Although he would not engage in direct play with me, Ricky did stand by and watch with a slight smile on his face as I rolled the ball to Maurice, who bounded back and forth, retrieving and barking. Occasionally, Ricky made further eye contact with me on his own effort, smiling as he did so. But he said nothing further.

After a few moments the boy fished a broken water pistol in the shape of a tiger from the toybox. He told me he was going upstairs to fill it with water. He ran up the basement stairs, opened the door at the top, and closed it rather loudly behind him. Then, a second later, he opened it and peered down at me at the bottom of the steps. "You can come up here and watch me if you want to," he said. But before I could join him at the sink in the bathroom, Mrs. Swartz gathered me up in a controlling way and directed me to a snack she had prepared for herself and me at the table in the family-room end of the large country kitchen. "Now," she said, "you'll have a chance to stop playing with Ricky and sit here and enjoy the nice, cozy fire. I've fixed us some coffee and cake." As she poured my cup, Mrs. Swartz continued, "You'll notice, over the hearth, the picture Ricky drew in kindergarten this morning. That one, scotch-taped to the mantel." She called Ricky into the room and told him to tell me a story about his drawing. Ricky came in, looked at the drawing, then silently spun on his heel and went back into the bathroom where he had been trying to fill the water pistol.

With tension in her voice, Mrs. Swartz took down the drawing, brought it to me at the table, and said, "I think it's excellent. Ricky has such creative talent in art, we think. Don't you agree?" Before I could answer, she said: "There, look under his name. He's spelled out the word s-e-v-e-n. I think that's marvelous—spelling so well, and a word so close to Kathy's age! Why, I think he just adores his bigger sister! But he wouldn't tell me the story that goes with these markings he's made on the other side. Ricky dear, won't you please come here and tell mother the wonderful story that goes with the other part of your picture?"

Ricky came in, all right, but not in a manner at all pleasing to his mother. He approached her and mumbled something unintelligible at first. Then, speaking clearly, he faced his mother with the angry comment: "Maurice bad dog! He bit my tiger [the water pistol]! Now it won't hold water. He's a mean dog! I'm going to burn him in the fire! I'll put him in the popcorn-popper!" Ricky ran over and picked up a long-handled popper beside the hearth. "I'll roast him in the fire until all the bite is out of him!"

Mrs. Swartz again attempted to spread saccharine denial over this very clear, nonpsychotic portrayal of his angry feelings by Ricky. "Oh, dear boy, why don't you come over here and show Dr. Looff your nice drawing. But first, you can put dear, sweet puppy outside." In an aside to me, Mrs. Swartz went on: "You know, Maurice and Ricky are inseparable. They have such lovely times together." At this point Ricky came over to his mother and muttered something about wanting to "listen to Ho-Ho." Mrs. Swartz looked relieved as she explained to me, "Music is another one of Ricky's creative things. He thinks about music all of the time. That's his name for 'Hi-Ho, It's Off to Work We Go'—you know, the song the dwarfs sing in *Snow White*. Well, Ricky has this perfectly lovely Walt Disney record. Let's all go in the library, and I'll put it on the machine for him. Ricky can't touch the machine —can you, Ricky? You see, Dr. Looff, it's a new stereo my husband just purchased and we don't allow the children to touch it." Gathering us up, Mrs. Swartz led the way into the library where she put on this particular record for Ricky.

In the twenty minutes that followed, Ricky smiled a great deal as he marched and danced there in the room as this record played. Once he asked me directly if I liked a particular song. "If you do, Dr. Looff, sing it, whistle it, and snap your fingers to it!" I did all three things with him, which delighted him. Once he allowed me to join hands with him as we danced around in a ring. At one point, when he was dancing alone, Ricky's heel caught the end of the new record-player cabinet. The jarring made the stylus jump. Momentarily alarmed, Ricky froze in his tracks. He turned an anguished face to me. As I said I didn't think he'd hurt the machine or the record, really, he relaxed somewhat. But he would not resume his dancing. Instead, he came over to the couch on which I was sitting and listened to the remainder of the record. I told him that I was glad to see him today, that I was pleased I could know his different feelings about his dog and about music. Mentioning my own children by name, I told him that our dogs, Charlie and Alice, did things at times that angered John and Mary. I told him how angry Mary had been when Alice chewed up a collar Mary had bought for her one Christmas, and how mad John was when Charlie chewed holes in a pair of his tennis shoes in our basement. Ricky watched me intently as I talked, but he said nothing.

At this point, the record had just gone off. Ricky asked me to turn it over for him. As I was intently studying the changer mechanism to accomplish this (my thoughts seriously occupied with the task of not damaging Mr. Swartz's stereo), Ricky stood beside me. All at once he reached up, drew his hand slowly down over my face, and said, "Make a smiling face." I began to learn from this event how carefully Ricky could observe others, and how he could often correctly infer others' true feelings from their nonverbal behavior. Generally, in the Swartz home, words covered rather than revealed feelings. What was so prominent there, that afternoon, was the fact that Ricky had not altogether abandoned the struggle to express his own feelings, or to know the real feelings of others. To be sure, he had allowed his mother to control many of his actions, and he had acceded somewhat to her denial of his feelings over his dog, for example. But he had not given up altogether in his attempts to define feelings accompanying events.

Just then, Kathy returned from school. As she burst through the front door, she spotted me in the library with Ricky. "Oh," she said, "you must be that child psychiatrist who's come to study the queer goings-on of my younger brother! He's really quite messed up sometimes, you know." There was a quality of the dramatic little actress in Kathy, I felt. She came over, looked at the record jacket lying on the rug, and held it up. Ricky jumped up angrily. "That's mine! You let me have it back!" Teasingly, Kathy held it over her head and told her brother, "Now, now, Ricky. I just want to read Dr. Looff all of the names of the songs you're listening to."

Drawn by this hubbub in the library, Mrs. Swartz came in from the kitchen in time to catch Kathy's last remark. "Well, dear, why don't you sit next to Dr. Looff on the couch and read him something from your school books. Really, Dr. Looff, Kathy is a marvelous reader. And she draws very well, too, for a child her age. You remember, Kathy, that you told me you wanted more than anything else to be a reader when you grow up! But you also told me you wanted to be an artist, too!" Kathy rolled her eyes and wriggled in delight at having her mother's exclusive attention. While this scene was going on, Ricky went over to the record player, hung his head over the cabinet, and seemed absorbed in watching the record go around. At this point, Mrs. Swartz complained, "That's what he's always doing. He becomes preoccupied and won't take any interest in what others are doing or saying!" In a moment, Mrs. Swartz and Kathy excused themselves and left the room. Ricky then turned to me and with obvious anxiety said, "I hate her sometimes!" Then, before I could respond, he told me with the same anxiety in his voice something about "my big sister, Marsha, who lives next door with Cheryl. Marsha likes me and comes over here to play with me a lot. I like her most of all!"

Later, Mrs. Swartz, who had overheard Ricky telling me this, explained that he had seen a picture of a University of Kentucky student named Marsha in the newspaper several months earlier. This girl in the newspaper photograph resembled Cheryl, the nineteen-year-old daughter of their neighbors. "Ricky seems to have fallen in love with Cheryl," Mrs. Swartz said. "He talks about her and Marsha all the time. But he won't actually play with Cheryl or speak to her in person." Shortly after this, our home visit was ended.

There in the Swartz home that afternoon, I had found Ricky capable of beginning to relate with me—genuinely, even if tentatively. Furthermore, he had shown that in spite of his problems in interpersonal relationships, he wanted very much to understand his own feelings and those of others. And he was able to begin using our relationship to talk about some of these feelings. In addition, Mrs. Swartz had shown some real feelings of her own—anxiety, dismay, even anger at one point—that had not been revealed earlier, in her office interviews.

As indicated earlier, such home-visit data were not necessary to round out our diagnostic impression of Ricky as a borderline psychotic child, or to enable us to see Mrs. Swartz as a woman who used denial of feelings to the point of significantly distorting Ricky's relationships with her and with others. But the data obtained that afternoon were crucially important to us in determining some important strengths both the child and his mother possessed as well. In time, they were able to allow these strengths in themselves to be tapped in therapy.

The reader may conclude from the examples given here that such additional methods or techniques as the utilization of picture albums, baby books, home movies, and home visits by the evaluator are best employed in instances where a psychotic or a borderline psychotic child is being studied. It is certainly true that our understanding of such children is augmented considerably by these procedures, but the same methods can apply to any child for whom certain features of the family's functioning remain obscure to us in our regular evaluation interviews.

Chapter 10.

Concluding the Evaluation

As explained in Chapter 2, the six-interview diagnostic study ends with a follow-up conference between the evaluator and the parents of the child. This important conference is, however, only one of the three parts of the final phase of the evaluation. These three parts are:

(1) Formulating the comprehensive diagnosis.

(2) The follow-up conference itself.

(3) Notification of the appropriate persons of the findings of the study and of the evaluator's recommendations for treatment.

In this chapter we examine each of these steps. To begin, we can readily see the relationship among them by referring again to the Russell family. We pick up their story at the point where members of the family have met with me in five diagnostic interviews. To summarize: Mrs. Russell had telephoned me initially about the problems she and her husband were having with seven-year-old Charlie. Following her inquiry, Tom and Alice Russell had talked with me in an initial joint interview that focused on the boy's current, visible problems, his ways of coping with conflict, and his strengths. Later, in individual interviews with them, I came to know more about Charlie's parents as people, and how in important ways each contributed to their son's growth as social models. In meeting twice with Charlie himself, I had these same themes rounded out for me through the boy's own understanding of himself. Special tests had been given. I had been able to obtain a recent school report directly over the telephone from Mrs. Snyder, Charlie's second-grade teacher. Finally, my talk with the boy's pediatrician had confirmed his parents' impression that he had been a healthy youngster all along. We were now at a summing-up point. In a follow-up conference, the three of us would pool our emerging thoughts and feelings

about the boy. We would talk over Charlie as we all saw him.
And we would plan toward whatever might be indicated for
his further care. Suggestions for conducting such conferences
are also given here.

Prior to the conference with Mr. and Mrs. Russell (step 2
above), I had to think through the various data that had
emerged from our interviews and pull everything together by
compiling a comprehensive clinical-dynamic-genetic diagnostic
formulation of the boy's problems and assets (step 1). Finally,
the third step that must be taken at the end of the evaluation
is to inform (by telephone and written summary letters) the
people who are in charge of the child's further growth about
the findings of the study and to explain the recommendations
for treatment. We now examine each of these steps in turn.

THE DIAGNOSTIC FORMULATION

Diagnosis is first a clinical-dynamic evaluation or a current
cross-sectional formulation of the child's presenting problems
in their total context. Such a statement includes an assessment
of (1) the area of conflict and the degree of the disability,
(2) the environmental stresses, (3) the strengths of the child
and his family, and (4) the specific ego patterns the child uses
in his current relationships with others. Thinking through the
diagnostic data to arrive at such a view of the child's total
functioning is the first step the evaluator takes. Although
there are several aids to preparation of this statement, one
that has served me well in my clinical work, the reader will
recall, was given in Chapter 1—a seventeen-point list of ego
functions. This list, as I indicated earlier, has served me in two
ways: First, it outlines the factors to be considered in data
collection during the diagnostic process. Secondly, it has afforded me a shorthand way of thinking through, and of writing up, this first part of the diagnostic formulation.

Specifically, I used this list of seventeen ego functions to
guide my writing of the "Clinical-Dynamic Summary" section
of the report on Charlie called *The Psychiatric Examination
of the Child* (see Appendix). Earlier, I had summarized the
data concerning background history and feelings obtained

from my meetings with Charlie's parents in the report called *History and Current Setting of the Diagnostic Study* (see Appendix for the form outline for such a report). And I had summed up the data from my two interviews with Charlie himself by writing them down in the first part of *The Psychiatric Examination of the Child*. In the clinical-dynamic summary section of this latter report, therefore, my cross-sectional view of Charlie's current ego functioning was as follows.

"Charlie Russell, the seven-year-old son of white, upper-middle-class parents, is a boy with probably bright normal to superior intellectual capacity. He is a sturdy, healthy, well-developed youngster. His motor movements are purposive and coordinated; there are no indications of neuromuscular problems; and special screening tests indicate he has no perceptual-visual-motor deficiencies. A warm, personable boy, he is essentially well-related with his parents, his younger sister, other adults (including this examiner), and children younger than himself, with whom he is inclined to be controlling and directive. Although he is initially liked by children his own age, his need to take over a group frequently brings him into aggressive conflict with other would-be leaders. His speech functions are excellent: he articulates well; he has an advanced vocabulary and a fund of general information well above age level; he uses language meaningfully in social discourse; and he is very capable of discussing his ideas and feelings with others.

"At times he can be very emotionally labile—his feelings of momentary anxiety, anger, disappointment, and sadness can erupt in intense ways that bring him into conflict with others. Such labile feelings produce, at times, periods of hyperactivity, shortened attention span, and, occasionally, explosive aggressive assaults on others or negative attention-getting behavior. At other times intense feelings of pleasure-in-mastery of some performance or intellectual task are equally labile, causing him to erupt into take-over-the-group leadership behaviors. In these ways the boy has a very real problem in acquiring and utilizing a well-modulated expression of emotional reactions to the environment.

"Generally, the boy's self-esteem is high; only momentarily, as when he is guilty over an aggressive outburst, is his self-concept diminished. His intelligence, which makes it easy for him to master many performance tasks requiring good visual-motor skills and school-type tasks well above his age level, strongly contributes to his high self-esteem. Along with his other good perceptual-cognitive capacities, his reality testing is well developed. His habit patterns of eating and excretion, of regular cycles of sleep and wakefulness, and of capability to engage in a variety of self-help tasks are age-appropriate.

"Through his general conduct and observable feelings of guilt and shame occurring after transgressions or lapses, the boy shows evidence of age-appropriate acceptance of prohibitions and sanctions, prevailing family and community customs, and ideas of decency. Although he currently fails to complete many of his second-grade assignments, there is strong evidence to suggest that the boy is acquiring formal elements of education more rapidly than his peers: he reads, retains, and comprehends written material up to a sixth- or seventh-grade level (school report and Gray Oral Reading Test); his spelling skills are at a third- or fourth-grade level (school report), and he makes good phonetic attempts at spelling more difficult words; and his arithmetic skills are at a third-grade level (school report).

"His adaptive, integrative ego strengths are several. He is a high-drive, rather intense, competitive, achievement-oriented youngster on the whole who enjoys meeting and mastering tasks in which he is interested. If he is not interested in a task (as with many school assignments), he loses any interest rapidly, becoming bored and restless. He has an excellent capacity for understanding and synthesizing the thoughts and feelings connected with events—including an excellent capacity for self-observation. However, his capacity to store tension is variable and, at times, momentarily deficient to the point that he cannot set effective inner controls over the eruption of his feelings. At such times he becomes easily frustrated, cannot store the tension his feelings engender, and acts out these feelings immediately, without delay or regard for the consequences. It is probable that this variability (at times deficiency) in his capacity to store tension accounts, in part, for his problems with emotional lability. At times, however, he can sublimate aggressive impulses into fantasy (the watered-down picture, for example) or into more socially approved outlets (dart-gun play, sports). His memory functions, both recent and remote, are good.

"The boy has a strong view of himself as a growing boy. Furthermore, his preoccupation with age-appropriate phallic-aggressive interests expressed in games, in his reading, and in fantasy suggests that he has no problems in basic psychosexual identification or in acquiring appropriate gender-role behavior. His basic life-style or personality structure is essentially normal. However, two elements of his life-style are contributing to the difficulties he is currently having with storing tension, with setting inner controls over aggressive-impulse pressures, and with emotional lability (his main current conflicts). One element is his congenital activity type[1] (gained from his developmental history) as a boy who from birth was somewhat hyperactive, irregular, intensely reactive, approaching, at times nonadaptive, inclined to have a low stimulus threshold, variable in mood, nonselective, and distractible. The other element in his life-style is a more recent one, a trend toward the development of an overly independent trait in his personality that makes disciplining the boy difficult at times for others. These two elements represent the internal factors the boy brings to his current conflicts over his aggressive-impulse pressures. His predominant defensive or coping techniques brought to bear on such conflicts are (1) maladaptive defenses: direct acting out of aggressive impulses (seen in aggressive assaults on others, and in negative, attention-getting behaviors); or occasional use of turning anger against the self (producing mildly self-destructive biting or destruction of his own possessions); and (2) more adaptive defenses: occasional suppression (patience-evoking maneuvers), sublimation (socially approved aggressive games), and discharge in fantasy."

Such a clinical-dynamic cross-sectional view of any child's current functioning, as indicated earlier, is arrived at by the evaluator's thinking through the diagnostic data. He summarizes the material in a manner that gives him an accurate, operational view of the child's functioning. Obviously, such a description is much more than the mere labeling of clinical signs and symptoms. These are included in the summary, of course, but symptoms are best understood as the product of the child's conflicts and attempts to cope with them. Thus

1. Stella Chess, Alexander Thomas, Herbert Birch, and M. Hertzig, "Implications of a Longitudinal Study of Child Development," *American Journal of Psychiatry, 117*, 1960, p. 434.

conflicts and defenses must be outlined in the summary as well. But more than that, if an ego-function approach is taken as a way of describing the child (the seventeen-point list used in this book is one example), symptoms, conflicts, and defenses are brought together into a more understandable picture of the child's functioning.

After he completes the ego-function summary of the child, the evaluator is in a position to make both (1) *a clinical diagnosis*, that is, a clinical classification of the child's disabilities or psychopathology, and (2) *a personality diagnosis* which describes the life-style of the child with a suitable term or phrase. Earlier, in the Preface of this book, I mentioned that I have found the nosological classification outlined in the *Group for the Advancement of Psychiatry Report No. 62*, "Psychopathological Disorders in Childhood: Theoretical Considerations and a Proposed Classification," very useful in my clinical work with children. Since 1966, when this proposed classification first appeared, I have taken my clinical diagnoses from it. Charlie's clinical diagnosis, from this text, was taken from the broad psychopathological category of developmental deviations. Specifically, his diagnosis within this group was "deviation in integrative development." This term was chosen to label Charlie's moderate deviation in development of the capacity to store tension and to develop tolerance to frustration. The boy's personality diagnosis was "essentially normal personality structure, with a recent trend toward developing an overly independent personality trait." These two diagnoses were recorded just under the clinical-dynamic-summary section in *The Psychiatric Examination of the Child* (see Appendix) of my final written report covering Charlie's evaluation.

As the next part of his thinking through and recording the complete clinical-dynamic-genetic diagnostic formulation for a particular child, the evaluator sums up the psychological, social, cultural, and biological-constitutional factors that, taken together, have through the years shaped the child's behavior. In effect, the evaluator now sums up the entire relevant field of forces or factors that have contributed in some measure to this shaping process. He examines the causal aspects of the longitudinal factors affecting the child's current behavior. From his diagnostic data, he interprets the reasons why the child responds now as he does and where and how his problems originated. These longitudinal factors are recorded together under "Genetic Factors in the Diagnostic Formulation." This phrase constitutes a heading for the appropriate section in the outline for *The Psychiatric Examination of the Child*. In my thinking through and writing up this particular part of my diagnostic formulation of Charlie's evaluation, I listed my conclusions about the genetic factors operating in his life as follows.

"1. *Biological-constitutional factors.* From birth, the boy's congenital activity type amounted to a deviation in sensory development. He had difficulty in monitoring sensory stimuli as shown by unusual sensitivities to certain colors and through difficulties in screening out certain stimuli (visual, tactile, social). At times he was clearly stimulus-bound, unable to sort out and relegate certain impressions to the background of a given experience; in effect, he had to take in and react to nearly everything in his environment at once. This led him frequently to respond overreactively to ordinary sensory input by becoming easily overstimulated. His manifest behavior, then, in response to this central problem in monitoring stimuli was hyperactivity, a poor attention span, and emotional lability. Thus his problem in monitoring stimuli later made it difficult for him to develop a full capacity to store tension. His history of ongoing development seems to indicate, however, that with the passage of time this deviation in sensory development is improving. It does not, at the present time, exert the same influence on his behavior as it did during his infancy and toddler periods of development.

"2. *Family factors.* Mrs. Russell was in a difficult emotional position at the time of the birth of her son and for the ensuing two or three years. Isolated from her family, having no friends in their new job location, finding no physical and emotional support from her husband, and criticized by both her mother-in-law and her husband for her at times inept handling of their son, Mrs. Russell became confused, anxious, frustrated, and somewhat depressed. Although she continued to function reasonably well in her mothering role in spite of these dysphoric feelings, Mrs. Russell defensively adopted a pattern at times of avoiding painful feelings by withdrawing from Charlie. Specifically, in later years she often gave up attempting to furnish the external controls the boy clearly needed at times when his inner controls over his aggressive impulses were lacking. Doubt over her ability to discipline her bright, impulsive son led her frequently to give up trying.

"Mr. Russell, for his part, has had until recently a tendency to face problems in his environment somewhat passively. For example, he is now aware that he has avoided assisting his wife in the past with their son's discipline. Reinforcing this personality trait in himself, for the first three years of their son's life, was his absence from home during that period (several jobs at once; exhausted when finally home).

"3. *Sociocultural factors.* Being shunned by his peers, who at times are driven away by his take-over, aggressive behavior, has had a negative, reinforcing effect on the boy's self-image to some degree. Missing, therefore, have been many opportunities for the boy to learn further control of his aggressiveness through the social give-and-take possible if he were an accepted member of a cohesive peer group.

"Important, too, in the present crisis over the boy's aggressiveness at school are factors operating both in the classroom situation and in his teacher. His second-grade class is quite large, and therefore his teacher cannot give him the individual attention that would positively lead him into special projects commensurate with his superior intelligence. Then, too, his teacher demands quiet in her classroom at all times and brooks no interference with her lesson plans. It would seem, in such a situation, that her life-style and the boy's are prone to clash."

THE TREATMENT PLAN

As the final part of the process of thinking through the diagnostic study of a child, the evaluator records his ideas of an ideal treatment plan for the child and his family. Here the evaluator makes his statement of recommendations regarding the nature of appropriate therapy. For example, he may recommend psychotherapy or drug therapy or a combination of the two; he may favor certain psychotherapeutic approaches —say, insight-producing or ego-supportive or crisis-oriented

psychotherapy; he may spell out appropriate behavioral modification approaches, preferring individual rather than group
or family therapy, a team of therapists rather than only one,
and so on. Also, the evaluator makes a realistic statement of
the goals of therapy (symptomatic relief versus personality
reorganization, degree of possible realignment of family balance, and so forth). Similarly, the evaluator records any special cautions or contraindications that he feels exist in connection with any particular treatment approach.

It is axiomatic that planning for comprehensive treatment
evolves directly from the preceding diagnostic formulation,
which gives purpose and direction to the therapeutic goals,
prognostic speculations, and plans to ameliorate or correct
the child's emotional disability. The plan will vary depending
on the child's needs and the family relationships and poten-
tialities as well as on the resources within the community.
The choice of professional personnel to carry out the treatment plan requires consideration of the training experience,
skills, and personalities of the persons available to perform
such treatment.

In sum, then, ideal treatment goals and methods are planned
individually for each child and his family according to the
specific diagnostic formulation. In each instance, the evaluator
attempts to devise specific treatment measures. Sometimes,
however, the treatment plan of choice cannot be put into
effect because of limited community, clinic, and personal staff
resources. In this event, an alternative plan with a more limited
goal may have to be followed. *It is important, however, that
the evaluator construct and record an ideal treatment plan
whenever possible* along with the reasons which necessitate
the adoption of a less desirable plan of action. This procedure,
in itself, will foster the development of diagnostic skills, sound
judgment, and flexibility.in treatment planning.

The individual treatment plan the evaluator devises may
include a variety of direct and indirect methods. Occasionally
only one type is indicated, centering primarily on physical,
psychological, or social factors. For example, the treatment
for one child with a learning problem is the direct treatment
of his visual defect; for another it is direct work with the
child in remedial reading; for a third it consists of an indirect
environmental approach by effecting an appropriate grade

placement in school; while for a fourth it consists of psychotherapy to alleviate the underlying neurotic learning inhibition. More often the plan of action involves both indirect and
direct procedures and deals with multiple interrelated facets
of the child's personality and his environment. For a child
with primary mental retardation, for example, the treatment
plan may encompass direct medical treatment, specialized education with vocational training either while he is living at
home or is in institutional placement, and perhaps psychotherapy to help the child resolve some of his inevitable worries and concerns. It also includes work with the parents, often
social casework services, to help them with their feelings in
the situation and to prepare them to take the next planning
steps.

Indirect treatment of the child solely through casework or
psychiatric treatment for the parents is frequently the pre-
ferred plan when the child's anxiety has not yet been internalized and when his problem occurs as a reaction to the parents' inappropriate attitudes and methods of child care. Such
a reactive disability may represent prolonged or exaggerated
conflicts specific to a particular developmental stage which
the child has difficulty in resolving because of the parents'
illogical attitudes and feelings. For these children, treatment
is geared to helping the significant parent, or both parents, to
understand the developmental problem and to handle it more
constructively. This method is often effective in dealing with
the problems of the very young child, but a favorable outcome
depends on an accurate evaluation of the parents' capacity to
modify their interactions with the child.

When a child has developed marked internalized, or intra-
psychic, conflicts and emotional disabilities that cannot be
alleviated by parental treatment alone or by some other environmental modification, the treatment plan includes direct
psychotherapy for the child. Depending on the nature and
degree of the child's psychopathology and strengths, varying
intensities of therapeutic work in particular areas of conflict
might be indicated. The specific psychotherapeutic methods
may range from supportive relationship therapy alone to
several kinds and levels of dynamic insight therapy. They may
be planned to emphasize one or more aspects of the treatment process: the abreaction of feeling while the child is

revealing directly or symbolically his conflicts and defenses; the working through of inner conflicts within the relationship with the therapist by the development of some insight through the clarification of dynamic patterns and the interpretation of genetic factors; and the strengthening of ego functions through reeducation, identification with the therapist, and the ultimate resolution of illogical attitudes in the therapeutic relationship.

Regardless of its level or intensity, effective psychotherapy for the child requires the participation of the parent or parents. For example, the achievement of continued masculine development in a passive, inhibited boy depends largely upon concomitant help for the parents in overcoming their restrictive, infantilizing attitudes as the child himself is helped to become more active. This collaborative parent-child treatment plan is a frequent one of choice for many troubled children and their parents. In many clinics or private practice settings, work with the parents may be done by the psychiatric social worker, by a clinical psychologist, by a psychiatric nurse, by a mental health associate, or by a psychiatrist. The prognosis in collaborative treatment is largely determined by the flexibility and strength of the several family members who are involved in the treatment plan, but it also depends on the skills of the professional persons involved and on the opportunity they have to work closely together in integrating their cumulative insights and developing their methods and goals in the continuous diagnostic-treatment process.

Occasionally the parents' active participation in a collaborative treatment process is contraindicated because of their lack of motivation and capacity to change or because changes might in fact be detrimental to the child's or the family's welfare. This occurs when parental patterns protect them from psychoses by maintaining some equilibrium, albeit pathological, within the family. In these instances, direct psychotherapy with the child alone has a very poor prognosis. Even if accompanied by attempts to foster healthier identifications and improved adaptations outside the family, direct psychotherapy still demands an unreasonable degree of self-sufficiency on the part of the child. Moreover, significant improvement in the child might seriously disrupt the tenuous family balance. Although older adolescents can occasionally be helped without the continued active participation of the parents, this is rarely if ever true for the younger child, whose further development still depends largely on his parents. Even with adolescents in the less seriously disturbed families, parental interest and support and at least their willingness to go along with the treatment plan are required.

When intensely disturbed family relationships prevent the child and parents from engaging constructively in a collaborative treatment process, the child's separation from the family is sometimes recommended as a temporary measure to facilitate treatment opportunities for both the child and his parents. This might involve, for example, a year of boarding school for a younger adolescent, while simultaneously both he and his parents are seen in psychotherapy and social casework. Or, as a necessary adjunct to psychotherapy, the child may require a corrective living experience in the therapeutic milieu of an inpatient psychiatric treatment facility. Some parents, relieved of the burden and stress involved in the everyday care of the disturbed child, have greater energies and motivation to face their own involvements and to modify their responses to the child. Inpatient psychiatric treatment for the child, with actively participating parents, facilitates the development of sound parent-child collaborative treatment. The goal is the child's return to his own home in a happier, more stable family relationship that will foster his continued emotional growth.

When parents lack the capacity or motivation for participation, the child's placement outside the home might be recommended in order to offer him a more supportive environment and the opportunity to benefit from such other treatment measures as might be indicated. The placement recommendation should be based on the child's particular needs. It should indicate whether a foster home, boarding school, resident school, special type of inpatient psychiatric unit, or other institution is desirable. Only too frequently, unfortunately, a specific plan cannot be carried out because of the dearth of appropriate facilities, and often the parents are unable to accept separation from the child. At all times, collaborative work in preparing the child and parents for placement is the ongoing responsibility of the persons who evaluated the family, in cooperation with appropriate community agencies. Sometimes when placement is more desirable but cannot be effected, the diagnostic formulation offers some reasonable basis for trying the traditional methods of outpatient collaborative treatment. At other times it is folly to proceed with treatment while the child remains in the home. In extreme situations when the child's welfare demands placement outside the home, it may be necessary to bring the child's plight to the attention of the official child welfare agency or court.

Other social modifications are frequently recommended as major or adjunctive aspects of a treatment plan. Diagnostic study may reveal that the child's disability represents a direct reaction to parental anxieties associated with difficult experiences such as financial insecurity or serious family illness. In such cases the treatment plan is geared to the correction of the family problem by referral to appropriate community resources. At other times children themselves are helped through environmental modification with or without direct pyschotherapy. Community recreational facilities, organized club activities, and day nurseries offer normal group experience and opportunity for developing skills and healthy behavior patterns. Special educational facilities are sometimes indicated. Teachers serve as significant adult figures for the child. Moreover, their observations of child behavior can be helpful to the persons involved in treatment, who in turn offer them support and understanding of the child's problems.

My conclusions about the ideal treatment plan for Charlie were recorded under the section entitled "Treatment Recommendations" at the very end of the report covering his evaluation. These were as follows.

"1. Charlie Russell's feeling-oriented verbal skills, his strong desire to have the social approval of adults around him, and his excellent capacity for self-observation combine to make him try out new approaches to his problems suggested by others. Already, during this evaluation, the boy has responded positively and more adaptively to more directed support given by his father and to some of the suggestions I have made to him. In these ways the boy shows a good capacity for further growth through learning and for further secondary socialization. He should, therefore, benefit from brief-contact, ego-supportive psychotherapy aimed (1) at strengthening his capacity to store feeling-engendered tension, and (2) at training him simultaneously in more socially approved ways of handling his intense feelings. Concurrently, joint counseling with his parents seems appropriate to reinforce their present desires to redirect their training efforts with their son by helping them use methods more conducive to the boy's acquiring inner impulse controls and safer ways of expressing his feelings.

"2. Ideally, the boy should be in a smaller class in which he can receive more individualized attention, in order (1) to avoid frustration by encouraging growth in school-type tasks commensurate with his superior intelligence, and (2) to provide an atmosphere mixing firm, kind, consistent limit setting, flexibility, and encouraging supports for learning.

"3. Psychotropic drugs do not seem indicated at this time. Other support measures are not required in the community at this time."

THE FOLLOW-UP CONFERENCE

The vital next step in concluding an evaluation and in treatment planning is the joint discussion with the child's parents of what they and the evaluator have learned during the diagnostic study. The child himself is usually not included in the follow-up conference. Instead, the findings of the evaluation and the treatment recommendations are discussed with the child in an individual interview, usually during the first treatment session, in a way he can understand at that time. Thus the follow-up conference represents a time when both parents and the evaluator—and any other collaborators who have been involved in the study—meet again to sum up their thoughts and feelings about the child. Overall, the follow-up conference includes an appropriate explanation of the clinical findings and recommendations summarizing the diagnostic study, as well as a review of the understanding which the parents may have gained about themselves, especially in relation to their children, as the interviews have proceeded. Insights acquired by the parents during the course of a diagnostic study often have a significant therapeutic potential. This was certainly true for the Russells, for example. However, most parents require further help in clarifying their motivations or in overcoming their resistances to the recommended treatment plan. At this point we shall consider some methods the evaluator can use to facilitate the movement within the conference and some general suggestions for conducting such a meeting.

First of all, *the evaluator can anticipate how the parents will feel and respond in the conference from the manner in which they have conducted themselves in the earlier interviews.* Their relationships with each other, and with the evaluator, have by the time of the follow-up conference established a kind of predictive utility. In effect, we have as evaluators found out during the course of the diagnostic study how much the parents are aware of the clinical-dynamic situation in the family and what their attitudes and feelings toward their child and his problems are. The predictive utility of this awareness is that we can anticipate what information the parents are ready to accept in the follow-up conference and make constructive use of, and we can guess how they will react to the measures suggested for helping their child.

Furthermore, *the evaluator who has been interviewing somewhat resistive parents all along has been working with the troubled feelings underlying these resistances,* In Chapter 4, for example, several types of feeling-based resistance were mentioned that usually occur during the initial, joint interview with the parents. Described there as well were ways the interviewer can accept, universalize-generalize about, reflect back, accurately label, and often enable the parents to work through the troubled feelings they may have. The point was made there that the goal of the evaluator throughout the diagnostic study is to provide the understanding support required to enable the parents to express the negative feelings which might otherwise have blocked their participation in the study. Having already helped the parents deal somewhat with their own anxieties and misconceptions, the evaluator has laid the groundwork of the kind of relationship—a working alliance— on which acceptance of his final summary statements and recommendations in the follow-up conference depends. Conversely, if he has not helped the parents deal with their troubled feelings earlier in the diagnostic study, their acceptance of the evaluator's statements at the time of the follow-up conference has been impeded, if not completely blocked.

With Tom and Alice Russell, the relationship was a true working alliance, and our discussion during the follow-up conference was quite productive. No major resistances were encountered. Alice Russell felt both informed and relieved when the factor of Charlie's congenital activity type, and the role it played in his past and present functioning, was gone over in some detail. "I feel so much better to know there was something different about him that made him hard to handle from the start. But I'm just as relieved to hear from you, Dr. Looff, that he really doesn't have minimal brain damage or something else like that." The remainder of my clinical-dynamic-genetic formulation was gone over with them in the same detail. Not feeling defensive, the couple were able to hear, understand, and begin to make constructive use of this explanation of Charlie's difficulties and assets.

For his part, Tom Russell was an active contributor to the conference. Feeling supported by his wife and by me for his recent efforts in steering Charlie away from a situation which might have been an occasion for an angry explosion on the boy's part, Tom reported that he planned to watch for further instances where he could help out. Charlie's educational needs were discussed as well. Moreover, both parents felt comfortable with the short-term, ego-supportive psychotherapy plan I outlined for the boy, with concurrent joint meetings with both of them planned as well. We decided that I would talk further with Charlie one hour a week initially, spacing our interview to every other week at a later date after his impulse controls were more firmly established. We also agreed that I would meet with both of them on a weekly basis to discuss— as we had already begun to do—how they could redirect their training efforts with Charlie. And, finally, we felt it would be appropriate for me to talk by telephone with Mrs. Snyder, Charlie's teacher, to review the findings of the evaluation and to assist her in planning his further school program. At my request, Mr. Russell signed a release-of-information form giving me permission to send a letter summarizing the findings of the evaluation both to the school (for inclusion in the boy's confidential file there) and to his pediatrician (for his general medical record).

As would other evaluators of children, I found it gratifying during the comprehensive diagnostic study of Charlie Russell to work with a family so essentially well-related, verbal, feeling-oriented, insightful, and cooperative. Such families are not uncommon in clinic and private-practice settings. Other families, of course, are much more conflicted than the Russells. For them the follow-up conferences may, at many points, hit snags of negative feelings. Progress is impeded until the evaluator has helped them deal with these feelings sufficiently to enable them to move on.

It is crucial that the evaluator be alert to these natural points of feeling-based resistance that many parents show. These resistances may come up quite openly, through angry negation of some of the points the evaluator is attempting to make, or through continued display of frustrated, angry, disappointed feelings toward the child himself. But sometimes resistances are more covertly displayed. For example, the evaluator may become aware in the conference that the parents are blocking out, failing to hear his statements. In either case, he realizes that he cannot continue attempting to summarize the findings of the evaluation.

Instead, he thinks through to himself just how it is that the parents' feelings have brought them to this point of resistance. He is aided in this understanding, of course, by his prior knowledge of each parent's personal background, of his or her lifestyle, and of the individual ways each parent—from his or her history—has come to feel about the child. Our primary concern as evaluators—certainly here, at resistance points blocking progress of the follow-up conference, but also during the major part of any diagnostic interview—has to be with the parents' feelings. For until these have been recognized, reflected, labeled, and dealt with, the parents are not in a position to accept a different view of their child—the dynamic view accounting for his particular behavior.

The evaluator can often help the parents recognize and deal with feeling-based resistances by sharing stories about the child's behavior. In other words, the evaluator shares with the parents his own natural feelings (raised, but not overreacted to) stemming from the child's behavior when he was alone with the evaluator in his diagnostic interviews. For example, one oppositional child, Susan, an adopted girl of twelve, often left me feeling frustrated and annoyed when she frequently blocked out, failed to hear, and tuned me out in our individual

interviews. During the follow-up conference, her parents—
whose life-styles encouraged the natural emergence of many
guilty feelings—blocked at the point where I had begun discussing some of the factors that, in my judgment, led to their
daughter's need to be so oppositional. I had begun to mention
parental overcontrol as a major factor. Both parents sat tight-
lipped and silent at this particular point. Obviously, it would
have been fruitless for me to pursue the discussion further.
Instead, I told them, in considerable detail, how frustrated
and annoyed I had felt inwardly when Susan tuned me out
on one occasion. I let my frustration and anger show a bit in
the follow-up conference. Almost immediately, Susan's
mother crackled: "There, you see. She does you the same
way! It makes me so damn mad when she pulls that same thing
on me! Drives me up a wall! Why can't she be quiet and dutiful, and do what I tell her to, like other girls I know?"

Susan's father joined his wife and me in agreeing that he
was made angry at times by their daughter's behavior. Then,
with anger released and labeled, they went on to say that they
had felt criticized by my earlier remarks, as though I were
blaming them altogether for the child's oppositional behavior.
Because they saw I could be angry, too, they felt supported—
the psychiatrist was saying he was in a similar spot with the
girl. The criticism could therefore be shared, they now felt.
My anger, in effect, had given them permission to open up
with theirs.

From here they went on to say, with real feeling, how much
they as parents of an adopted child wanted to do an adequate
job in their parenting role. But the harder they tried (overcontrol), they said, the more stubborn Susan seemed to become. This made them feel guilty and ashamed, as though
they were failing as parents. This guilt was the feeling, we
were then able to conclude, that had quickly surfaced to
cause their silent resistance when I had begun to point out
how they might have contributed to the child's behavior.

To sum up this technique, I would label it *a personal sharing of quite natural feelings the child's behavior evokes in the
evaluator* which serves, through a permissive and universalization-generalization approach, to put the evaluator and the
parents in the same boat. In these resistant situations, the
evaluator's sharing of his feelings about the child's behavior

often creates quick empathy. The evaluator is no more or less human than themselves, the parents see. This frequently makes it possible for him to encourage the parents to express their troublesome feelings more directly. The parents then simply follow the example of the evaluator, who was saying clearly how he had felt in a somewhat similar situation with their child. The evaluator then accepts the direct expression of the parents' feelings, thereby dissipating some of their intensity. After this has happened, and the parents have been assured of the competence and interest of the evaluator (this assurance itself is fostered by the evaluator's working alliance with the parents), they are generally ready to understand their child in different, dynamic terms.

The Three-phase Approach. Thus I adopt a three-phase approach to the conduct of follow-up conferences concluding diagnostic evaluations of children.

(1) The first phase involves the evaluator's accurate understanding of and appropriate reflection of parents' feelings, attitudes, and expectations toward their child. It is essential for these feelings to be identified and, to some extent, worked through. Failure to do so blocks the progress of the next phase.

(2) This phase involves a mutual discussion between the evaluator and the parents leading to a fuller, more accurate, dynamic understanding of the child's total functioning. As this discussion proceeds, some part-functions of the child are described as relatively conflict-free, and the mentioning of these generally evokes no negative feelings from parents. However, as in the instance of my attempt to discuss Susan's behavior in more depth, some functional areas in the child are charged, for the parents, with tremendous emotion. Emerging dysphoric feelings block their further participation in a dynamic discussion at just these points. Then the evaluator is called upon to double back, to do some more first-phase work as it were, to enable the parents to join him again in the dynamic discussion. This moving back and forth between phases, this ebb and flow, is common in follow-up conferences.

(3) The third phase, which logically proceeds from the other two, involves the mutual discussion of the many, often collaborative aspects of treatment planning. The parents and the evaluator can at this juncture begin to discuss methods that

will help them deal with their child more effectively at home. This three-phase conceptualization of the natural progress of follow-up conferences can serve us usefully in our clinical work.

SUMMARY REPORTS

Planning treatment for the child also includes making recommendations to the referring person or agency. This communication—by telephone, initially, followed by a summary letter—is a basic responsibility of the evaluator. Contact by telephone is personal, permitting mutual discussion between the evaluator and the other person that summary letters alone can never provide. Using this approach (a telephone call followed by a letter) facilitates the development and maintenance of good working relationships with people who not only refer children for evaluation and treatment but also have an important, ongoing part to play in their further growth and development. School personnel, of course, are an obvious example of those who are immediately concerned with the children we evaluate and who, therefore, need our immediate feedback at the end of a diagnostic study.

In my telephone conversation with Mrs. Snyder, Charlie's second-grade teacher, for example, both of us had an opportunity to clarify our collaborative roles in his ongoing care and education. Mrs. Snyder welcomed my formulation on the whole, and was pleased that I would be seeing all members of the family in treatment interviews. Most important of all, however, was her own awareness of the part she and her classroom situation contributed to shaping some of Charlie's school behavior at the present. "Dr. Looff, I can see Charlie got along fine with you in a one-to-one situation. But in my classroom, with thirty-two youngsters to teach, I don't have the time to give him the individual attention I know now he needs. Besides, I'm rather fixed in my ways. I need order and quiet to teach effectively. And Charlie's never going to fit that bill. We both see that. So I think it would be best, all in all, if he were shifted out of my class to Miss Jones's second grade. She's got a smaller, experimental group this year, and she is very enthusiastic about bright, challenging children. At the same time, she is a limit-setter. I've felt all along, and you've confirmed it now for me, that Charlie would do better under her for the balance of this school year. If you like, I'll talk with the principal and Miss Jones about this. Will you talk with Mr. and Mrs. Russell about it for me?" Just as Mrs. Snyder had carefully worked it through in her own feelings and insights, her suggested school plan proved to be, in time, an effective one for Charlie. With my call to her, and after my summary letter was sent subsequently to the school (with a copy to the pediatrician), the diagnostic evaluation of Charlie Russell and his family was completed.

CONCLUSION

In this book I have discussed ways of approaching children and their parents who come to us for diagnostic evaluation of their troubled feelings and behavior. These families are asking us for help. Much of this book has underscored the extent to which the evaluator reaches out to and shares himself with the children and their parents. In natural ways this sharing begins and deepens the relationship the evaluator builds with them. This relationship, first and foremost, is the cornerstone of the working alliance that those who evaluate families hope to construct as evaluation proceeds. Much of the rest of the book has involved the enumeration and explanation of interview techniques that one can use to facilitate the flow of diagnostic interviews once beginning relationships have been established with the child and his parents.

Overall, the book has focused on ways we as evaluators can assist families in trouble. Often their calls for help must be painstakingly deciphered in the home and in our offices before they can become the basis for positive, joint action. The rewards are profound. When progress begins during the diagnostic study, and we are relating to and working with children and their parents in this kind of joint endeavor, we see them beginning that extraordinary experience which all people imbued with new hope undergo—the flowering of their inherent capacity to grow and develop.

Appendix

DEVELOPMENTAL QUESTIONNAIRE

Identifying Information

1. Child's Name _____
        First   Middle   Last
   Birthdate _____ Age _____ Religion_____

2. Child's Address _____
       Number and Street   City and Zip Code
   County _____ Telephone_____

3. Natural Father's Name _____
       First   Middle   Last
   Birthdate _____ Age _____ Religion _____

   Place Employed _____ Position _____ Hours _____

   Home Phone _____ Work Phone _____

4. Natural Mother's Name _____
       First   Middle   Last
   Birthdate _____ Age _____ Religion _____

   Place Employed _____ Position _____ Hours _____

   Home Phone _____ Work Phone _____

5. Date of Marriage _____

6. If Divorced, Date of Divorce _____

   If Remarried, Date of Remarriage _____

   Step-Parent's Name _____
       First   Middle   Last
   Birthdate _____ Age _____ Religion _____

   Place Employed _____ Position _____ Hours _____

   Home Phone _____ Work Phone _____

DEVELOPMENTAL QUESTIONNAIRE (Cont.)

7. Living in home with child:

Mother _____
       Name   Age   Legal Relationship

Father _____
       Name   Age   Legal Relationship

Others _____
       Name   Age   Legal Relationship

        _____
       Name   Age   Legal Relationship

        _____
       Name   Age   Legal Relationship

        _____
       Name   Age   Legal Relationship

        _____
       Name   Age   Legal Relationship

8. Child's brothers and sisters living outside the home:

        _____
       Name   Age   Occupation

        _____
       Name   Age   Occupation

        _____
       Name   Age   Occupation

        _____
       Name   Age   Occupation

        _____
       Name   Age   Occupation

9. If child adopted, give date of legal adoption _____

10. Name of child's school _____

    Name of teacher _____

    School grade _____

    School address _____

11. Referred to Child Division by _____
                                      Full Name

    Address _____ City _____

DEVELOPMENTAL QUESTIONNAIRE (Cont.)

12. If child has been seen at any other agency:

Name of Agency _____ For Purpose of: _____

_____ _____

_____ _____

13. Previous Psychiatric Examinations and Treatment of Patient:

14. Describe the Current Problem As You See It:

DEVELOPMENTAL QUESTIONNAIRE

To Be Filled In by Parents

Patient's Name _____ _____ Date _____

1. Was the child planned?

2. What was the mother's health during the pregnancy with the patient:

   (a) Was she nervous and apprehensive; unusually happy; moody; other reactions. Describe.

   (b) Physical condition: Headaches, high blood pressure, and/or pus in the urine; any special medical conditions.

   (c) Was she taking medicine while she was pregnant? If so, what?

   (d) Nausea, vomiting; persistent abdominal or lower back pain; spotting; excessive fatigue? Duration?

   (e) Illnesses of any kind: Flu, virus infection, measles, or others? Temperature? Dates and duration of illness.

   (f) Any accidents or falls? Describe.

3. What were the mother's activities during pregnancy?

DEVELOPMENTAL QUESTIONNAIRE (Cont.)

4. Did the mother feel that the living situation or events in the home were comfortable during this period? Describe.

5. What was the father's attitude toward the mother being pregnant? Describe.

6. Approximately how long was the mother in labor? _____ hours. Was labor difficult or easy? _____ Was labor induced? ____ Were forceps used? _____ Other. Describe.

7. Was father at the hospital during birth of the child?

8. What was father's attitude toward the birth of the child? Describe.

9. What part of the baby was born first? Head _____ Buttocks _____

10. Weight of baby at birth _____. Was he full-term? _____ If not, how much earlier or later than the expected date did the baby arrive?

11. Did the baby breathe spontaneously and easily? _____ Did he need oxygen and other medical assistance after delivery? If yes, what?
_____
_____

Was there anything exceptional in the baby's condition such as injury, paralysis, blueness, excessive crying? Explain.

12. Did the mother have convulsions, hemorrhages, infections, unusual nervousness, tears, or anything else at or soon after childbirth? Explain.

DEVELOPMENTAL QUESTIONNAIRE (Cont.)

13. Was the baby breast-fed? _____ Bottle-fed? _____ Or received both types of feeding? _____

   (a) If combined feeding, at what age was transfer from breast to bottle made? _____

   (b) If bottle-fed, were there difficulties in finding a suitable formula? _____ Describe: _____

   (c) If breast-fed (partially or completely), did the mother experience any difficulty with: Scanty milk supply, nursing painful, cracked or inverted nipples, etc. Describe. _____
   _____
   _____

   (d) Does the mother recall the baby's response to nursing? Active _____ Eager _____ Had to be encouraged _____

   (e) What were the mother's feelings about the nursing experience? Describe. _____
   _____

14. Which type of feeding was used? _____ Demand _____ Time schedule? _____
   _____

15. When the baby vomited, was he apt to bring up his food in small amounts, or did it come up in large quantities and with force? Describe.
   _____
   _____
   _____

16. Were there times when the baby had frequent spells of colic, constipation, or diarrhea? _____ At what ages? _____ How was it handled? _____
   _____

17. What attitude or mood did the baby seem to express most of the time? For example: Happy; smiling and laughing; "cuddly"; whining; seemed in pain; sad; "old"? Describe. _____
   _____

DEVELOPMENTAL QUESTIONNAIRE (Cont.)

18. Did anyone assist the mother in the care and responsibility of the baby during infancy? _____

19. Generally, babies vary in regard to the amount of activity they show. Which of the following do you think would most nearly describe your baby during the first few months of his life:

    (a) Showed a great deal of activity such as squirming, wiggling, kicking, and otherwise moving about so that it caused concern or difficulty, etc. _____
    _____

    (b) Showed very little physical activity, not even showing any increase in movement, interest, or response when hungry or when played with. _____
    _____

    (c) Showed vigorous activity when awake and when played with but was equally often observed playing quietly and generally relaxed.
    _____

    (a) _____ (b) _____ (c) _____ (d) Other (Describe):
    _____
    _____

20. During the baby's first year of life was there anything (even if it had nothing to do with the baby) that caused unhappiness or anxiety, or placed the mother or father under special strain? Describe. _____
    _____
    _____
    _____
    _____

21. Each child has his own individual sleeping pattern. Describe some of your child's sleeping habits, such as: Thumb-sucking, rocking, requiring a special toy, blanket, or other object. _____
    _____
    _____

DEVELOPMENTAL QUESTIONNAIRE (Cont.)

22. Did the baby sleep alone in a room? _____ If not, with whom did he share it? _____ At what age? _____ For how long a period? _____ Did the baby sleep alone in a bed? _____ If not, with whom did he share it? _____ At what age? _____ For how long a period? _____

23. Were there any periods when the child habitually awoke crying and any periods in which he had to be held or rocked in order to fall asleep? _____ At what age? _____ What else would soothe or quiet the child? Describe. _____
    _____
    _____

24. How old was the baby when he was able to sit up alone for a sustained period of time? _____ Stand? _____ Crawl? _____ First steps? _____ Walk unaided? _____. Did he have difficulty in achieving any of these? Describe. _____
    _____
    _____

25. At what age did the baby first speak a few isolated words, such as da-da, ma-ma, bye-bye? _____ Speak in simple phrases? _____
    _____

26. Did your child have any difficulty in learning to talk? _____ At what age? _____ Describe. _____
    _____
    _____

27. How old was the child when toilet training was started? _____

    (a) What methods were used? (State whether child was placed on a receptable or "toidy" seat; how frequently; how long he was left there; what was done if the child was unsuccessful; whether enemas or suppositories were used; whether he cried or struggled.) _____
        _____
        _____

DEVELOPMENTAL QUESTIONNAIRE (Cont.)

(b) Were training methods made difficult for any physical reasons, such as constipation, diarrhea, etc.? _____

_____

_____

(c) At what age was bowel control established? _____ Were there any relapses, and under what circumstances did these occur? At what ages? _____

_____

_____

(d) Does the child soil at this time? _____

28. What training methods were used to teach the child bladder control?

_____

_____

(a) At what age did the child stop wetting himself at night? _____

(b) At what age did the child stop wetting himself in the daytime? ____

(c) Were there any relapses? _____ At what age? _____

(d) Does the child still wet himself? _____

29. What were the child's reactions and attitudes toward toilet training?

_____

_____

_____

30. What were the child's and the parents' reactions to thumb-sucking; masturbating; nail-biting?

	Child	Parent
Thumb-sucking		
Masturbating		

DEVELOPMENTAL QUESTIONNAIRE (Cont.)

	Child	Parent
Nail-biting		

31. Has the child ever had angry outbursts, temper tantrums, or other kinds of behavior which caused you concern? Describe. _____

    Under what circumstances did they seem to occur most frequently?

32. Has the child ever screamed? _____ Stomped? _____ Thrown things? _____ Thrown himself on the floor? _____ Hurt others? _____ Hurt himself? _____ Held his breath? _____ Banged his head on things? _____ Withdrawn? _____ Describe the physical appearance of the child during these periods. _____

    Did he seem to know what he was doing? _____ How early did they occur at first? _____ At what age did the child have them most frequently? _____ How often did they occur? _____ At what age did they stop? _____ By whom were these handled: By mother? _____ By father? _____ By nursemaids? _____ By others? _____

33. What methods have you used in disciplining?

    Spanking   _____

DEVELOPMENTAL QUESTIONNAIRE (Cont.)

Withholding of privileges _____

Withholding of approval and show of affection _____

Others—describe. _____
_____
_____
_____

(a) How does the child respond to discipline? _____
_____
_____
_____

(b) Has discipline been frequently necessary? _____
_____
_____
_____

(c) Who ordinarily disciplines the child? _____
_____
_____

34. Have the parents and/or relatives agreed with each other on methods of discipline and privileges or have there been disagreements? Describe.
_____
_____
_____

35. During the early years of the child's life, was either parent frequently away or out of the home? (Business trips, hospital, military service.) Describe. _____
_____
_____

36. Has the child ever expressed fear of: darkness, dogs, trains, etc.? Or had frightening dreams? _____ At what age? _____ Did these fears cause any special problems? Describe. _____
_____
_____

DEVELOPMENTAL QUESTIONNAIRE (Cont.)

_____

_____

_____

_____

_____

_____

37. Has the child ever had daydreams, fantasies, or imaginary companions?
At what age? _____

Daydreams _____

Fantasies _____

Imaginary companions _____

38. Has the child ever lost any person with whom he seemed to have a close relationship, such as father, mother, sister, brother, grandparents, or others? At what age? _____ Who? _____ Explain. _____

_____

_____

39. Has the child ever seemed reluctant to be left in the care of others, or objected to it? Describe. _____

_____

_____

40. Did the child have any preschool or school experiences such as nursery or kindergarten in which separation from home was difficult for him?

_____

_____

41. Currently, does he prefer playing with children of his own age? _____
Older? _____ Younger? _____ One or two friends? _____
Many of them? _____ Are his friends among his own social group

DEVELOPMENTAL QUESTIONNAIRE (Cont.)

or children the parents did not expect him to choose? _____
_____
_____

42. Does the child seem to have a closer attachment to one parent than the other? _____ Which one? _____ Were there any changes in his attachments, and, if so, when did they occur? _____
_____
_____
_____

43. Has the child ever required his parents or others to do things for him which he was capable of doing for himself? Describe. _____
_____
_____
_____

44. Has the child ever had strong likes and dislikes for food? _____
_____
_____

45. Has the child ever had any frightening experiences? Describe the experience, his age and his reaction. _____
_____
_____
_____
_____

46. How was the child prepared for the birth of brothers and sisters? _____
_____
_____
_____

By whom? _____ How did he respond? _____
_____

47. Did he show marked preferences or dislikes for any of his brothers and sisters? _____ How was this expressed? _____
_____
_____

DEVELOPMENTAL QUESTIONNAIRE (Cont.)

How are these feelings expressed currently? _____
_____
_____
_____

48. Has the child shown curiosity in regard to the origin of babies? _____
At what age? _____ What is his understanding of this? _____
_____
_____
_____
_____

49. Was the child prepared for menstruation? _____ At what age? _____
At the onset of menses was she shocked? _____ Tearful? _____
Casual? _____ Pleased? _____ Indifferent? _____

50. At what age did your child begin school? _____ If he began later than
six, why? _____
_____

51. Has your child ever been retained in one or more grades? _____ If so,
which grades? _____

52. Has your child ever skipped one or more grades? _____ If so, which
grades? _____

53. Does your child spend a lot of time studying? _____

54. What are his study habits? Discuss briefly. _____
_____
_____

55. Circle the word or words which best describe(s) your child's grades
throughout his school experience.

Superior.   Above average.   Average.   Below average.   Failing.

DEVELOPMENTAL QUESTIONNAIRE (Cont.)

56. In a few words, describe your child's attitude toward school when he first started. _____

_____

_____

What is his current attitude? _____

_____

57. Were there any attempts to change left-handedness to right-handedness?

_____

What attempts were these? _____

_____

Were they made at home? _____ At school? _____

58. Has the child ever had any motor coordination difficulties, such as confusion in regard to left-handedness or right-handedness, or frequent falling, awkwardness in throwing a ball or riding a bicycle, etc.? _____

_____

_____

_____

_____

_____

_____

_____

_____

_____

59. List illnesses the child has had. State age at which each occurred, how long each illness lasted, what treatment was given, and if there were any unusual reactions or after effects:

Illnesses	Age	Treatment Given	Reactions

DEVELOPMENTAL QUESTIONNAIRE (Cont.)

Illnesses	Age	Treatment Given	Reactions

If you need more space, please use the back of this paper.

60. Did the child have any operations such as: circumcision, tonsillectomy, adenoidectomy, etc.? State:

    (a) Age at which operation occurred.

    (b) Was child hospitalized, and for how long?

    (c) Was recovery uneventful, or were there complications such as vomiting, high fever, etc.?

Operations	Age	Hospitalization	Complications

What was child told about operation beforehand? _____
_____
_____
_____

DEVELOPMENTAL QUESTIONNAIRE (Cont.)

What reaction did child show afterwards, that is, fearfulness, temper tantrums, increased shyness? _____
_____
_____
_____

Child's attitude toward doctor before and after operation? _____
_____
_____
_____
_____
_____
_____
_____
_____
_____
_____
_____

61. What accidents did the child have and when? Describe, and state what happened and how child reacted. _____
_____
_____
_____
_____
_____
_____
_____
_____
_____
_____

DEVELOPMENTAL QUESTIONNAIRE (Cont.)

62. Is the child on any medication at the present time? _____
    If so, what kind and for what was it prescribed? _____
    _____
    _____
    _____
    _____
    _____
    _____

Signed: _____

BENDER SCREENING TEST DESIGNS

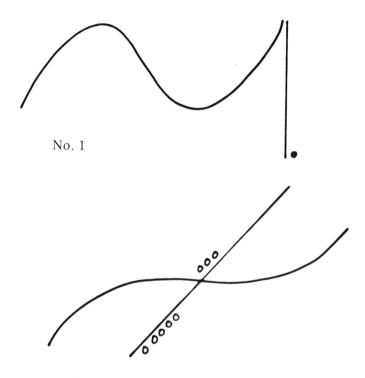

No. 1

No. 2

BENDER SCREENING TEST DESIGNS (Cont.)

No. 3

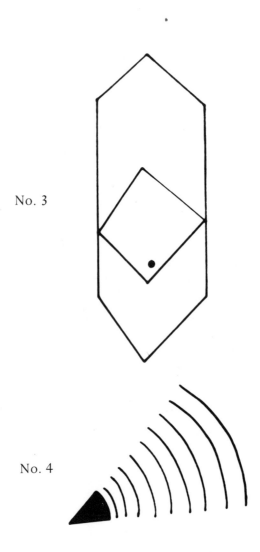

No. 4

GRAHAM-KENDALL SCREENING TEST DESIGNS

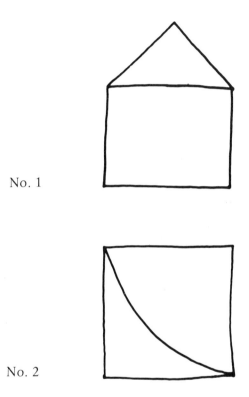

No. 1

No. 2

GRAHAM-KENDALL SCREENING TEST DESIGNS (Cont.)

No. 3

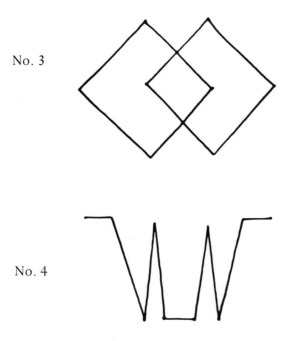

No. 4

THE DESPERT FABLES*

1. *The Bird Fable:*
   To ascertain whether there is a fixation to one of the parents or whether the child is independent.
   A Daddy and a Mommy bird, and their little baby bird, are asleep in the nest on a branch. But all of a sudden a big wind blows; it shakes the tree, and the nest falls on the ground. The three birds awaken all of a sudden. The Daddy flies quickly to a pine tree, the Mother to another pine tree. What is the little bird going to do? He knows how to fly a little already.

2. *The Wedding Anniversary Fable:*
   To ascertain whether the child may have witnessed sexual intercourse in the parents' room; jealousy toward parents' union.
   Daddy and Mommy are celebrating the day when they were married. They love each other and they have arranged a beautiful party. During the party, the child gets up and goes all by himself to the end of the garden. Why, do you suppose?

3. *The Lamb Fable:*
   To investigate the weaning complex and sibling rivalry.
   In a field there is a Mommy sheep and her little lamb. The little lamb bounces around all day near his Mommy. Every night his Mommy gives him some good warm milk, which he likes very much. But he can already eat grass. One day somebody brings to the Mommy sheep a tiny little lamb who is hungry, and he wants the Mommy to give him milk. But the Mommy sheep has not enough milk for the two of them; and she says to the bigger lamb, "I haven't enough milk for two; you, you are bigger, you go and eat some nice fresh grass." What do you think the bigger lamb is going to do? And how do you think he feels?
   (To investigate the weaning complex alone, do not mention the arrival of the little lamb; say that the Mommy sheep has no more milk and the lamb must begin to eat grass.)

4. *The Funeral Fable:*
   To investigate hostility, death wishes, guilt feelings, self-punishment.
   A funeral is going through a village street, and people ask, "Who is

* Reprinted with the Permission of the *American Journal of Orthopsychiatry.*

it that is dead?" Somebody answers, "It's somebody in the family who lives in this house." Who is it?

For the child who has no conception of death, tell the fable in the following way:

Somebody in the family took a train and went way, way, far away, and will never come back. Who is it? (Enumerate the members of a family.)

5. *The Anxiety Fable:*
Regarding anxiety and self-punishment.

A child says softly to himself, "Oh, I am afraid!" What do you suppose he is afraid of?

6. *The Elephant Fable:*
Examination of the castration complex.

A child has a little stuffed elephant which he likes very much, and which is very pretty with his long trunk. One day when he comes back from school, he comes into his room and finds that his elephant has changed. How do you suppose he has changed? And why is he changed?

7. *Fable of the Child's Own Creation:*
To test the possessive and stubborn complex (anal complex).

A child has made something with clay—a tower—which he thinks is very, very pretty. What is he going to do with it? His mommy asks him to give it to her. Do you think he is going to give it?

8. *Walking with the Father or Mother Fable:*
To detect the oedipus complex.

A boy went to the park for a nice walk with his Mommy. They had a lot of fun together. When he comes home, the boy finds that the Daddy's face doesn't look quite the same. Why?

Tell the fable for a girl in the following way:

A girl went to the park for a nice walk with her Daddy. They had a lot of fun together. When she comes home, the girl finds that the Mommy's face doesn't look quite the same. Why?

9. *The News Fable:*
To test the wishes and fears of a child.

A child comes back from school (or a walk), and his Mommy tells him, "Don't begin your homework right away, I have some news to tell you." What do you suppose the Mommy is going to tell him?

10. *Bad Dream Fable:*

    For a check on the preceding fables.

    A child wakes up one morning all tired, and he says, "Oh, what a bad dream I had!" What do you suppose he has dreamed?

NEUROLOGICAL EXAMINATION OF THE CHILD

	Ck if OK	Comments	If pathologic, record degree (Scale 1-5)

I. *GENERAL*

  A. Height, weight _____
     Head circumference

  B. Dysplastic appearance _____

  C. Neurological aspects
     of free play _____

    1. Maturational level _____

    2. Motor patterning

       a. General _____

       b. Fine finger coordination _____

       c. Handedness _____

    3. Anti-gravity behavior _____

    4. Pathological exploration
       (grasping, devouring, destroying) _____

    5. Impulsivity _____

    6. Unawareness of dangers _____

  D. Relationship with examiner

    1. Clinging, leaning,
       attempts-at-fusion _____
       Other motor dependency

    2. Response to handling-as-if-younger _____

    3. Clowning and other cover of disabilities _____

II. *MOTOR*

  A. Global or minimal findings

    1. Non-specific awkwardness

       a. Standing _____

       b. Walking _____

       c. Running _____

       d. Hop and skip _____

       e. Walk and run up and down stairs _____

       f. Catch and throw a ball _____

NEUROLOGICAL EXAMINATION (Cont.)

	Ck if OK	Comments	If pathologic, record degree (Scale 1-5)

g. Button and unbutton clothes _____

h. Tying shoes _____

i. Imitation of finger movements _____

j. Drawing _____

k. Writing, printing _____

l. Point at something _____

2. Associated movements

   a. Arm swing _____

   b. Eye, head, facial _____

   c. Articulation and phonation _____

   d. Speech with gestures and facial expression _____

3. Ability to dissociate movements (Eye, head, facial) _____

4. Extraocular movements in other non-test situations _____

5. Motor overflow; synkineses _____

6. Other adventitious movements _____

7. Suggestions of choreo-athetoid qualities _____

8. Suggestion of facial asymmetry _____

9. Speech

   a. Articulation _____

   b. Phonation _____

   c. Blending of articulation and phonation _____

B. Muscle tone

   1. Amount _____

   2. Quality _____

   3. Variability _____

C. Muscle strength: arms

   1. Amount _____

NEUROLOGICAL EXAMINATION (Cont.)

	Ck if OK	Comments	If pathologic, record degree (Scale 1-5)
2. Symmetry			
D. Muscle strength: legs			
1. Amount			
2. Symmetry			
E. Cerebellar function			
1. Romberg test: arms down			
a. Postural equilibrium			
b. Eyelid closure			
c. Eyelid fluttering			
d. Motor overflow phenomena			
2. Romberg test: arms forward, fingers spread, and counting to 25			
a. Elevation of arms			
b. Convergence, divergence of arms			
c. Convergence, divergence of fingers			
d. Eyelid closure			
e. Eyelid fluttering			
f. Motor overflow phenomena			
3. Whirling test, arms forward, fingers spread			
a. Shoulder rotation			
b. Trunk rotation			
c. Whole body rotation			
d. Elevation of arms			
e. Convergence, divergence of arms			
f. Convergence, divergence of fingers			
4. Tandem walking			
5. Toe-walking and heel-walking			
6. Stand on one foot			
7. Hop (in place) on one foot			
8. Finger-to-nose			

NEUROLOGICAL EXAMINATION (Cont.)

	Ck if OK	Comments	If pathologic, record degree (Scale 1-5)
9. Finger-to-finger			
10. Heel-knee-shin			
11. Rapid alternating movements			
a. Forearm pronation-supination			
b. Thumb-to-fingers			
c. Foot-tapping			
d. Tongue			
12. Fine coordination of fingers			
13. Rebound phenomena			
14. Nystagmus			
a. Resting position			
b. Extreme lateral gaze: left			
c. Extreme lateral gaze: right			
d. Extreme upward gaze			
e. Extreme downward gaze			
15. Tremor			
a. Rest			
b. Intention			
c. Both			

III. *SENSORY*

   A. Discriminatory sensation

      1. Topognosis (point localization—touch a spot on the child's body while his eyes are closed. Child then opens eyes and attempts to point to the exact point stimulated. Record number of errors in 1st and 2nd runs).

	1st Run	2nd Run
Rt. great toe		
Lf. knee		
Lf. thigh		
Rt. abdomen		

NEUROLOGICAL EXAMINATION (Cont.)

	1st Run	2nd Run
Lf. wrist		
Lf. shoulder		
Rt. wrist		
Lf. abdomen		
Rt. shoulder		
Lf. forehead		
Rt. forehead		

2. Double simultaneous stimulation, homologous (same region)
2. Double simultaneous stimulation, heterologous (different region, ipsilateral part contralateral)

1st and 2nd runs consist of 10 trials each. Tell child he may be touched in one or two places. Eyes closed. He tells the examiner the number of places touched. Then he opens eyes and points to where he was touched. Feet (F) and wrists (W) points of stimulation.

	No. of errors; region	
1st Run	perception extinct	2nd Run
LF & LW		RF & RW
RF & LW		RF & LF
RF & LW		LF & RW
RF & RW		RF & LW
RF & LF		RW & LW
LF & LW		LF & LW
LF & RW		RF & LF
RW & LW		RF & RW
LF & RW		RW & LW
RW & LW		LF & LW

	Ck if OK	Comments	If pathologic, record degree (Scale 1-5)
3. Two-point discrimination (Use distal phalynx of middle finger of rt. and lf. hand. Record in mm shortest distance between the points at which the child recognizes the two stimuli as distinct)			

NEUROLOGICAL EXAMINATION (Cont.)

	Ck if OK	Comments	If pathologic, record degree (Scale 1-5)

4. Stereognosis (Close eyes,
   identify: key, paper-clip,
   coin, button) _____

5. Graphesthesia (Palm of
   hand: write with key,
   etc. X, 0, B, D, 1, 6, 9)_____

6. Baragnostic sense (Dis-
   criminate gross and fine
   weights) _____

B. Non-discriminatory sensation

1. Proprioception (big toes and index fingers) (Close eyes—tell
   examiner if digits up or down)_____

2. Vibration (Use maximal bang C-128 tuning fork. Record
   qualitative response, i.e., "I feel it." Then record quantitative
   response, i.e., latency of response to off signal, wait 5 seconds,
   then record)

	Qualitative (On)		Quantitative (Off)	
	R	L	R	L
Maleoli				
Knee				
Iliac crest				
Wrist				
Elbow				
Shoulder				
Clavicle				

3. Touch (omit if topognosis is intact) _____

4. Pain (pin-prick: ask child to indicate if point or head, or sharp
   or dull)

	Right	Left
Legs		
Thighs		
Rt. and Lf. Abdomen		

NEUROLOGICAL EXAMINATION (Cont.)

	Right	Left
Thorax		
Neck		
Face		

5. Temperature (omit if pain sensation is OK) _____

6. Deep pressure _____

	Ck if OK	Comments	If pathologic, record degree (Scale 1-5)

IV. *CRANIAL NERVES*
II, III, IV and VI

1. Pupils R R & E _____

2. Pupillary reaction to light _____

3. Pupillary reaction on accommodation _____

4. Strabismus _____

5. Conjugate deviation
    a. Coordination _____
    b. Range _____

6. Convergence _____

7. Visual fields _____

8. Visual acuity _____

9. Color vision _____

V

1. Touch and pain sensation
    a. Face _____
    b. Scalp _____
    c. Ears _____
    d. Neck _____

2. Masseter and temporalis muscles
    a. Size and tone _____
    b. Symmetry _____

NEUROLOGICAL EXAMINATION (Cont.)

	Ck if OK	Comments	If pathologic, record degree (Scale 1-5)

V and VII

1. Corneal reflexes

   a. Briskness _____

   b. Symmetry _____

VII

1. "Show teeth" grimace _____

2. Puff out cheeks _____

3. Whistle _____

4. Raise eyebrows, wrinkle forehead _____

5. Squeeze eyes tight shut _____

6. Wink _____

VIII

1. Otoscopic examination _____

2. Hearing (by audiometer) _____

3. Weber (Place stem of 256 cycles/sec. tuning fork on child's occipital prominence or middle of forehead and record lateralization. If AC deafness is present, sound is lateralized to side of AC deafness and to the healthy side in the presence of unilateral nerve deafness) _____

4. Rinne (Place tuning fork on mastoid process until child no longer hears sound. Then the still-vibrating prongs are held opposite the auditory meatus. Normal AC is twice BC) _____

NEUROLOGICAL EXAMINATION (Cont.)

	Ck if OK	Comments	If pathologic, record degree (Scale 1-5)

IX and X

1. Palate position _____

2. Palate elevation _____

3. Gag reflex _____

XI

1. Trapezii: strength _____

2. Trapezii: symmetry _____

3. Sternocleidomastoids: strength _____

4. Sternocleidomastoids: symmetry _____

XII

1. Tongue: size and appearance _____

2. Tongue: adventitious movements _____

3. Tongue: voluntary movements _____

    a. Protrusion: position _____

    b. Protrusion: strength _____

    c. Push to right _____

    d. Push to left _____

4. Tongue: fibrillation; fasciculation _____

V. *MISCELLANEOUS*

  A. Identification of body parts

    1. "Point to your . . . " _____

    2. Topognosis (see sensory exam) _____

  B. Finger agnosia (touch finger while child has eyes closed. Then open eyes and ask child to indicate which finger touched) _____

  C. Right-left orientation _____

NEUROLOGICAL EXAMINATION (Cont.)

	Ck if OK	Comments	If pathologic, record degree (Scale 1-5)

D. Lateral dominance (handedness, footedness, eyedness)

    1. Report of the child _____

    2. Report of others _____

    3. Comb hair _____

    4. Reach for candy _____

    5. Reach for door-knob _____

    6. Wipe nose _____

    7. Throw ball _____

    8. Swing bat _____

    9. Aim toy rifle _____

    10. Kick _____

    11. Draw and write _____

    12. Ocular dominance _____

VI. *REFLEXES*

  A. Deep tendon reflexes (check as well for pendularity)

    1. Biceps _____

    2. Triceps _____

    3. Brachio-radialis _____

    4. Knee jerk _____

    5. Ankle jerk _____

  B. Cutaneous reflexes

    1. Abdominal _____

    2. Cremasteric _____

  C. Pathologic phenomena

    1. Clonus

      a. Ankle _____

      b. Patellar _____

NEUROLOGICAL EXAMINATION (Cont.)

	Ck if OK	Comments	If pathologic, record degree (Scale 1-5)
2. Plantar reflexes			
a. Babinski			
b. Gordon			
c. Chaddock			
d. Oppenheim			
e. Rossolimo's (tap ball of foot—positive if four toes flex)			
f. Mendel-Bechterew's (tap area in front of external malleolus—positive if there is flexion of the four toes)			
3. Hoffman (tap nail side of fingers—positive if thumb adducts)			
4. Tromner (tap palm side of fingers—positive if thumb adducts toward palm)			
5. Palmo-mental (elevation of chin)			

HISTORY AND CURRENT SETTING OF THE DIAGNOSTIC STUDY

Child's name _____Interviewer _____

Medical chart number _____ Dates of interviews _____

Identifying Information

Identifying data and description of the child, parents, siblings; name, age, race, religion, marital status and occupation of parents.

Source of Referral

Referral source and reason for present application. Previous help utilized (personnel, clinics, agencies, etc.).

History and Current Setting of the Presenting Problems

Informants: Description of each parent or other informant—their appearance and behavior. Evaluation of the reliability of each informant. If joint interview with parents or other caretakers, accurate description of modes of communication, relationship with the interviewer and with each other. Verbal and nonverbal cues. Insert waiting-room talk and behavior, other vignettes available.

Interview Content: Detailed history, with attendant feelings, of the presenting problems and strengths in the child as viewed by the informants. Dates and ages of the child during significant events. Relationships the informants have with the child; and the relationships the child has with all significant others. This is an intensive, searching, detailed historical inquiry into these areas. Record evidence the informants have of the child's varying feelings during these events.

Developmental History of the Child: Summarize here the significant events, delays in maturation, feelings related to task mastery or failure, and parental modes of training taken from the Developmental Questionnaire and from the informants' elaboration to the Questionnaire.

Recent School Report: Summarize data here obtained from the child's teachers.

Recent General Medical Report: Summarize here pertinent data obtained from the child's pediatrician or other physicians.

Family Setting and History

1. *Current family functioning:* characteristic parent-child and child-parent interactions. Child-siblings and siblings-child. Include family role behavior, social relationships, strengths in the child.

2. *Personal-social history of the father:* the background history of the father as it affects his parenting and marital roles.

3. *Personal-social history of the mother:* same considerations.

4. *Initial evaluation of parents' personalities:* their life-styles. Summary of each parent's contributions to the child's problems. Parental strengths, flexibility. Include here an initial evaluation of family dynamics: conflict areas and conflict-free spheres of functioning. Typical ways of coping with stress each parent has. Parental capacity for orientation to feelings, insight, motivation for participation in the child's care.

THE PSYCHIATRIC EXAMINATION OF THE CHILD

Child's name _____ Interviewer _____

Medical chart number _____ Dates of interviews _____

Identifying Information
Name, age, sex, mother and father, religion, siblings, birthdate, school and grade, teacher.

Source of Referral
Referral source and reason for present application.

Summary of Presenting Problems
Brief statement summarizing the present problems.

Interviews
A. *Appearance and behavior:* description of size, coloring, distinguishing physical traits, clothing, grooming. Posture and gait; gestures, mannerisms. Motor patterns (hyperactivity, retardation, tensions, inhibitions, distractibility, attention-span, etc.). Speech and thought disturbances (lisping, stuttering, stammering, pressured speech, use of pronouns-phrases-sentences. Looseness of associations, irrelevancy, incoherence, blocking, etc. Affective attitude (mood state: happy, sullen, apathetic, withdrawn, etc.). Manner of parent-child separation. Behavioral reactions of the child in terms of his relationship with the interviewer.

B. *Interview content:* child's understanding of his problems, strengths, characteristic ways of coping with stress; orientation of his feelings, capacity for insight are critically involved as the child relates his story. The child's awareness of his relationships with others, and the degree to which he sees himself as successful at mastery of various tasks. Review of the child's special interests, talents, hobbies, skills, goals.

C. *Special tests:* Gray Oral Reading Test. Graham-Kendall and Bender screening tests. Draw-a-person test. Time-spatial orientation. Neurological examination summary (if done). Other special tests (speech and hearing, etc.).

D. *Fantasy material:* Fantasy material as elicited through the Despert Fables, controlled and free-play situations, three wishes, rocket-trip-to-the-moon, animal-change, a million dollars, dreams and daydreams, early memories, drawings and associations to them.

Clinical-Dynamic Summary
A. *Summary of highlights* of interviews and observations organized according to the list of seventeen ego functions of the child (integration of findings of the psychiatric examination of the child with data of family and social, psychological, and physical and developmental studies into a comprehensive, working diagnostic evaluation). Formulation of current areas of conflict for the child and his family. Review of characteristic ways each copes with stress; conflict-free spheres of child and family functioning.

PSYCHIATRIC EXAMINATION OF THE CHILD (Cont.)

B. *Clinical diagnosis*—including any differential diagnosis.
C. *Personality diagnosis.*

Genetic Factors in the Diagnostic Formulation
Reconstruction of earlier dynamic-genetic factors and of multiple etiologies (current and past). Evaluation of ego strengths of the child and his parents. Evaluation of the readiness of the child and his parents for treatment. Evaluation of the significance of the diagnostic study to the child and his parents.

Treatment Recommendations
A. *Ideal plan* for comprehensive care and treatment.
B. *Modified plan* on practical basis of availability of treatment facilities, community resources, and the family's and the child's potential for participation in treatment.

Index

sex-role confusion. *See* psychosexual
development.
sexual development. *See* psychosexual
development
sexuality: crisis over, 25, 61; promiscuity, referral for, 16. *See also*
psychosexual development
sharing, personal, as interview technique, examples of, 114-15,
196-97
short-term treatment. *See* psychotherapy
sibling, older. *See* "predictor"
social data. *See* psychosocial data
social development, deviations in. *See*
"apron-string child"
social learning theory, orientation to,
6
social workers: as evaluators of children, 23; as therapists, examples
of, 34-38, 58. *See also* psychotherapy
socialization, 6
sociocultural factors in diagnosis, 186
socioeconomic data. *See* psychosocial
data
Southern Appalachian migrants, 7
Southern Medical Journal, 61
specific learning disabilities. *See*
learning disabilities
speech and hearing assessment, indications for, 12
Spock, Benjamin, 125
Stanford-Binet Test, 158
stealing, as crisis, 25, 61
structured play, use of, 153-54. *See
also* interviews; play materials
stubbornness. *See* oppositional behavior •
sublimation, capacity for, 8
subsistence farms, 55
suicidal attempts, as crisis, 25, 61
Sullivan, Harry, 15
summary statements, as interview
technique, 89, 120
superego operations, 8, 116
synthetic capacity, 8

task-mastery, capacity for, 8
task-oriented trade training. *See* vocational training
teachers: knowledge of children, 4,
16; and example of, 96-99;
preparation of children for calls
to, 76; and example of, 96-97.
See also schools
teasing. *See* peer group norms
techniques with children. *See* interviews
telephone reports. *See* agencies;

telephone reports *(cont.)*
physicians; teachers
television. *See* fantasy items
temper tantrums, case examples of,
54, 77, 120, 127
tension-storage, capacity for, 8
tests. *See* neurological examinations;
perceptual-motor functioning;
psychological testing; reading testing
Thematic Apperception Test, 147,
158-60
Thomas, Alexander, 183
"thousand dollars, finding a," as
fantasy item, 149
"three wishes," as fantasy item, 149
"three-phase approach, the," in
followup conferences, 197-98
Time magazine, 41
time-spatial orientation, testing for,
139-40. *See also* perceptual-
motor functioning; learning disabilities
training patterns, 6-7, 11; need for
redirection in, 54. *See also* cultural training patterns
transactions, interview, model for,
86. *See also* interviews
treatment planning, elements in, 186-
92
truancy. *See* schools

underachievement, classroom, example
of, 98
underemployment. *See* poverty
unfamiliar situation, fear of. *See*
separation anxiety
universalization-generalization: as
interview technique, 87-88, 114;
use of, 47, 51
University of Cincinnati, College of
Medicine, 27
University of Kentucky, College of
Medicine, 133, 155
University of Kentucky Medical
Center, 31, 50
unusual sensitivities in young children, 125

validation of feelings. *See* consensual
validation
value orientation. *See* superego operations
verbal communication. *See* language
skills
verbal skills. *See* language skills
visits, home. *See* home visits
visual-motor functioning. *See* perceptual-
motor functioning
vocabulary level. *See* language skills